War Wounds

Front cover photograph: Australian infantrymen evacuate a wounded soldier on a stretcher to the beach during the landing at Balikpapan, Borneo, July 1945. [AWM P04663.024]

War Wounds

Medicine and the trauma of conflict

edited by
Ashley Ekins and Elizabeth Stewart

EXISLE

First published 2011

Exisle Publishing Limited,
'Moonrising', Narone Creek Road, Wollombi, NSW 2325, Australia.
P.O. Box 60-490, Titirangi, Auckland 0642, New Zealand.
www.exislepublishing.com

National Library of Australia Cataloguing-in-Publication entry

Title: War wounds: medicine and the trauma of conflict / edited
by Ashley Ekins and Elizabeth Stewart.
Edition: 1st ed.
ISBN: 9781921497872
Notes: Includes bibliographical references and index.
Subjects: War--Medical aspects--Australia.
Medicine, Military--History--Australia.
Soldiers--Wounds and injuries--Treatment--Australia.
Other Authors/Contributors: Ekins, Ashley K. (Ashley Kevin)
Stewart, Elizabeth, 1964-
Dewey Number: 355.3450994
ISBN 978-1-921497-87-2

10 9 8 7 6 5 4 3 2 1

Text design and production by Janine Brougham
Cover design by Nick Turzynski, redinc.
Printed in Singapore by KHL Printing Co Pte Ltd

This book uses paper sourced under ISO 14001 guidelines
from well-managed forests and other controlled sources.

Contents

Korea

Vietnam

Personal stories

Preface

The history of warfare and the history of medicine have long been intertwined. Hippocrates of Kos, the ancient Greek physician who is generally considered the founder of Western medicine, even counselled aspiring young doctors to follow war as the only proper training for a surgeon. I understand this remains so today for trauma surgery.

During the twentieth century, wars resulted in many advances in medical treatment and surgery. Modern weaponry became more destructive and medical techniques and procedures were developed to deal with the massive scale and changing nature of battlefield casualties. A paradox also emerged: as war grimly expanded the opportunities for clinical research and the application of scientific discovery, developments in preventative medicine also increased the effectiveness of fighting forces through improvements in soldiers' health and disease resistance.

The major wars of the last hundred years—from the First World War to the recent and current conflicts in Iraq and Afghanistan—have driven advances in treatment for wounds and pain management, and more effective preventative measures against disease and infection. New approaches have been developed to evacuate, treat and heal the injured and wounded. Nevertheless, war continues to inflict its toll of carnage and human misery on not just combatants but also civilians who are, too often, either the intended or accidental targets of modern conflicts.

For veterans, and their families too, the post-war legacy of combat experience can sometimes seem as severe and persistent as the effects of wounds and injuries. The war-damaged soldier became a conspicuous figure in the aftermath of the First World War as repatriation agencies worked to alleviate the suffering of invalided veterans, to allocate appropriate pensions, and to introduce the first struggling medical recognition of the symptoms of deferred, post-traumatic stress.

In many respects, modern military medicine must remain equally concerned with treating the consequences of military service on veterans' health as with treating soldiers during their service.

These and many other aspects of the interaction of war and medicine are the primary themes of this volume. All the chapters were originally presented at an outstandingly successful international conference, *War Wounds: medicine and the trauma of conflict*, convened by the Australian War Memorial in September 2009 with the support of the Department of Veterans' Affairs and the involvement and interest of the Minister, the Honourable Alan Griffin MP, who kindly opened the event.

This conference attracted an eclectic and, as it turned out, dynamic mix of historians, medical practitioners, military medical officers, medics, nurses and veterans who explored the myriad experiences of casualties in war, their impact and aftermath, from their different perspectives. The event aroused considerable interest among the military, the public and the media, and undoubtedly led to a heightened general awareness of this important area of military-medical history.

Many moving personal stories also emerged as the lessons of the past served to illuminate problems of the present and to enhance understanding of veterans' issues and the enduring impact of war on Australian society.

The conference was originally conceived by Ashley Ekins, Head of the Memorial's Military History Section, who, with his colleague Elizabeth Stewart developed the program and jointly compiled and edited this collection. Each of them also contributed a chapter based on their own particular research interests. I acknowledge their dedication along with the contributions of the many fine scholars who participated in the conference and collaborated in the production of this book.

A number of other people contributed their skills and efforts. In particular, I thank Ian Watt and Benny Thomas and their team at Exisle Publishing for once again producing a high-standard publication that the Memorial is proud to sponsor. Among Memorial staff, Ron Schroer expertly administered the publication arrangements, editors Robert Nichols and Andrew McDonald edited the diverse collection of papers to the publisher's requirements, and Aaron Pegram of the Military History Section researched photograph collections and wrote many of the captions. Diane Lowther compiled the index.

Every effort has been made to locate current holders of copyright for text and illustrations reproduced here but we apologise for any omissions and would welcome information to enable amendments to be included in future editions.

One notable contributor was Professor Simon Gandevia who discussed his father's experiences as a regimental medical officer with an Australian infantry battalion in the Korean War. He also announced a generous family bequest to the Memorial to establish the Bryan Gandevia Award, an annual military history award in his father's name, to foster research among junior scholars into significant areas of military-medical history.

That award, this book, and the conference that inspired it, has demonstrated once again the Australian War Memorial's commitment to historical research and to maintaining the Memorial's pre-eminence as one of the finest research facilities in the world. As Professor Jay Winter of Yale University graciously noted in the introduction to his fine keynote address to the *War Wounds* conference:

> It is right and proper that we speak of a subject of the import-ance of war wounds here at the Australian War Memorial. This is where serious reflection on the Great War happens. Yours is a unique institution, braiding together the emotive power of a shrine, the representational power of a museum, and the scholarly riches of a great archive. After over 40 years of working in this field, I can say with some confidence that the Australian War Memorial is the premier centre for First World War studies in the world today. It enables scholars and laymen to come together in an act of recognition, the recognition that the Great War shaped the world in which we live.

Professor Winter's incisive comments might be applied to all major wars. His words should inspire and encourage future generations of scholars and soldiers not to forget 'the lessons of history'.

Steve Gower
Director, Australian War Memorial
May 2010

Notes on contributors

Jay Winter is Charles J. Stille Professor of History at Yale University. He is an internationally renowned scholar of the First World War and its impact on the 20th century. His interests range widely, including the remembrance of war in the 20th century, European population decline, the causes and institutions of war, British popular culture in the era of the Great War and the Armenian genocide of 1915. Professor Winter is the author or co-author of over a dozen books, including significant landmark works such as *The Great War and the British People* (1986), *The Experience of World War I* (1988), *Sites of Memory, Sites of Mourning: The Great War in European cultural history* (1995), and *1914-1918: The Great War and the shaping of the 20th century* (with Blaine Baggett, 1996). He has contributed more than 40 book chapters to edited volumes, and edited or co-edited 13 books including a collection of essays entitled *America and the Armenian Genocide*. His most recent publications include *The Great War in history: Debates and controversies, 1914 to the present* (with Antoine Prost, 2005), *Remembering war: The Great War between memory and history in the twentieth century* (2006), *Dreams of peace and freedom: Utopian moments in the twentieth century* (2006), and *Capital cities at war: A Cultural History* (2007). In 1997, Professor Winter received an Emmy award for the best documentary film series of the year as co-producer and co-writer of *The Great War and the Shaping of the Twentieth Century*, an eight-hour series broadcast on PBS and the BBC, and shown subsequently in 28 countries. He is one of the founders and a member of the comité directeur of the research centre of the *Historial de la grande guerre*, the international museum of the Great War, in Péronne, Somme, France. His next book is a biography of René Cassin, First World War soldier, humanitarian jurist and author of the Universal Declaration of Human

Rights, *René Cassin: Un soldat de la grande guerre* (forthcoming Fayard, Paris, 2011).

Ashley Ekins is Head of the Military History Section at the Australian War Memorial in Canberra. A graduate of the University of Adelaide, he specialises in the history of the First World War and the Vietnam War. He is the co-author (with Ian McNeill) of two volumes of *The Official History of Australian Involvement in Southeast Asian Conflicts 1948-1975* dealing with Australian army operations in the Vietnam War: *On the Offensive* (2003), and *Fighting to the Finish* (forthcoming 2011). He has published widely on the role of Australian soldiers in the First World War and contributed chapters to several books, including the volume he compiled and edited, *1918 Year of Victory: The end of the Great War and the shaping of history* (Exisle Publishing, 2010). He also contributed the introduction and supplementary material to *The Anzac Book* (Third edition, University of New South Wales Press, 2010). Ashley is currently completing a comprehensive study of military discipline and punishment in the Australian army of the First World War.

Kerry Neale is a PhD candidate at the University of New South Wales, Australian Defence Force Academy, Canberra. She is currently finalising her thesis, entitled '"Without the Faces of Men": the Experiences of Facially Disfigured Great War Veterans of Britain and the Dominions'. In 2009 Kerry was an Australian Bicentennial Scholarship holder at the Menzies Centre for Australian Studies, King's College, London. She is a graduate of the Australian National University, BA (Hons), and was awarded the University Medal in History in 2007. She was an Australian War Memorial summer scholar in 2006, and worked at the Memorial from 2004 to 2008 in the Visitor Services and Military History sections.

Marina Larsson is a Melbourne historian who has held lecturing positions at La Trobe and Monash universities. She is the author of the award-winning book, *Shattered Anzacs: Living with the Scars of War* (2009), a study which explores the impact of war disability on First World War returned soldiers and their families. In 2008, she received the Australian Historical Association's biennial Serle Award for the best postgraduate thesis in Australian History. Marina's research interests include repatriation history, disability history, public history, and the history of the family.

Paul Weindling is Wellcome Trust Research Professor in the History of Medicine at Oxford Brookes University. He has published *Health, Race and German Politics* (1989), *Epidemics and Genocide in Eastern Europe* (2000), *Nazi Medicine and the Nuremberg Trials* (2004) and *John W. Thompson, Psychiatrist in the Shadow of the Holocaust* (2010). He directs a project on victims of Nazi human experiments covering several thousand life histories of victims. He also researches physicians who were refugees from Nazism.

Debbie Lackerstein is a lecturer in history in the School of Humanities and Social Sciences, University of New South Wales, Australian Defence Force Academy, Canberra. Her teaching and research interests include the history of the Second World War, occupation and resistance, the Holocaust and genocide in the twentieth century. Her study of France in the 1930s and under German occupation, *National Regeneration in Vichy France*, will be published by Ashgate in 2011. Debbie is currently engaged in research into different perspectives on the liberation of the German concentration and labour camps at the end of the European war in 1945.

Simon Gandevia is a medical graduate and neurophysiologist. He is a founder and Deputy Director of the Prince of Wales

Medical Research Institute. He has received three research doctorates (PhD, MD and DSc), all from the University of New South Wales. His research focuses on how the human brain controls movement. Professor Gandevia's work has provided insights into pathophysiological mechanisms in several branches of medicine including neurology, rehabilitation and cardiorespiratory medicine. He has served on several editorial boards including for the *Journal of Physiology*, trained many doctoral students, and helped develop concepts about the ethics of experimental studies in humans. Professor Gandevia was elected Fellow of the Australian Academy of Science in 1998.

David Bradford is a sexual health physician, foundation fellow of the Australasian Chapter of Sexual Health Medicine and was made a Member of the Order of Australia for his services to sexual health medicine. He graduated from Sydney University in 1965. In 1967–68 he was Regimental Medical Officer (RMO) for 4 Field Regiment, Royal Australian Artillery, in South Vietnam. He studied surgery and obtained Fellowship of the Royal College of Surgeons in 1972. Later he was a general practitioner in the East End of London. On his return to Australia in 1979 he worked full-time as Director of the Melbourne Sexually Transmitted Diseases (STD) Clinic. He moved to Cairns in 1993 as Director of Sexual Health and since retirement in 2004 still conducts occasional clinics. David's book, *The Gunner's Doctor: Vietnam Letters* (2007) tells the story of his service in Vietnam in the form of letters home.

Elizabeth Stewart is a historian in the Military History Section at the Australian War Memorial. She worked for several years as a research officer on *The Official History of Australia's Involvement in Southeast Asian Conflicts 1948–1975* and from 2004–8 was content leader for the Vietnam section of the Memorial's Conflicts 1945 to today galleries. She is the co-author of two books (with Gary McKay): *Viet Nam Shots: A photographic account of Australians at War* (2001), and *With Healing Hands: the untold story of the Australian civilian surgical teams in Vietnam* (2009).

Graham Walker graduated from the Royal Military College, Duntroon, into the Royal Australian Infantry. He saw active service attached to the 2/7 DEO Gurkha Rifles in Sabah and Sarawak during the Indonesian—Malaysian Confrontation and with the 8th Battalion, Royal Australian Regiment in Vietnam where he was Mentioned in Despatches. Graham has been for many years the Honorary Research Officer of the Vietnam Veterans' Federation of Australia.

Peter Edwards is a consultant historian and writer, who has published on Australian defence and foreign policies for more than thirty years. He has held professorial positions at Deakin University in Melbourne, the Australian Defence Force Academy in Canberra, and currently at Flinders University in Adelaide. As Official Historian of Australia's involvement in Southeast Asian conflicts 1948–75, he wrote the volumes dealing with strategy and diplomacy, *Crises and Commitments* (1992) and *A Nation at War* (1997). He is also the author of *Arthur Tange: Last of the Mandarins* (2006), *Permanent Friends? Historical Reflections on the Australian-American Alliance* (2005), and *Prime Ministers and Diplomats* (1983); the co-editor of *Facing North* (vol. 2, 2003); the editor of *Australia Through American Eyes* (1977) and Arthur Tange's memoir, *Defence Policy-Making* (2008); and one of the founding editors of the series of Documents on Australian Foreign Policy. He is a Member of the Order of Australia and his books have won several literary awards.

Tony White was born in Australia but brought up in Kenya. He entered the Royal Australian Army Medical Corps as a medical student via the Undergraduate Scheme. After his intern year, he was posted to the 5th Battalion, Royal Australian Regiment, as RMO and saw active service in Vietnam in 1966–67. Subsequent postings included RMO to 1 Recruit Training Battalion, Kapooka, and to the British Military Hospital in Singapore. Following return to civilian life, he qualified first as a physician and then as a dermatologist. His appointments have included Visiting Medical Officer, Royal Prince Alfred Hospital, Clinical Senior Lecturer (University of Sydney) and Colonel Consultant Dermatologist, Army Office, Canberra. He is in private practice in Sydney and has a special interest in remote area dermatology, including the Pacific Islands and Arnhem Land. He does an annual circuit with the Royal Flying Doctor Service out of its Broken Hill base.

Sharon Cooper (now Sharon Bown) gained her Bachelor of Nursing degree at the University of Tasmania in 1995. After further study and work as a registered nurse, she joined the Royal Australian Air Force as a direct entry Nursing Officer in January 1999. Her first posting was to 3 Combat Support Hospital, Richmond, NSW. She deployed to East Timor in 2000 and again in 2004, when she was badly injured in a helicopter crash, suffering spinal injuries and facial fractures. Following 12 months of rehabilitation, Sharon returned to unrestricted service. She deployed again on Operation Bali Assist II in October 2005 to aid in the aero-medical evacuation of injured Australians following a terrorist bombing incident. Sharon was promoted Squadron Leader in 2007 and her recent roles have included a period as Aide-de-Camp to the then Minister for Defence, Dr Brendan Nelson, and a three-month deployment in 2008 to Tarin Kowt, Afghanistan, as the Officer in Charge of the Australian Medical Task Force providing intensive care and surgical support to the International Stabilisation Assistance Force – Afghanistan.

Graham Edwards served in the regular army for three years from 1968–71 and saw service in Vietnam with the 7th Battalion, Royal Australian Regiment in 1970. He was wounded twice in Vietnam, the second time losing his legs to a 'jumping-jack', anti-personnel land mine. After discharge from the army and a period of rehabilitation, he spent ten years with the Commonwealth Public Service in the Departments of Defence, Veterans' Affairs and in the Vietnam Veterans' Counselling Service. Graham was elected as a Councillor with the City of Stirling in 1980 and in 1983 was elected to the Parliament of Western Australia, where he served for fourteen years including seven years as a Minister. In 1998 Graham was elected to the House of Representatives in Federal Parliament where he served until he retired in 2007. He was recognised by the RSL with the Anzac of the Year award in 1991 for service to the veteran community; and he has also been awarded the Rotary Paul Harris Fellowship and the Lions Melvin Jones Fellowship. He is currently a member of the Prime Ministerial Advisory Council on Ex-Service Matters and a member of the Council of the Australian War Memorial.

Introduction

Elizabeth Stewart

On 24 April 2004 US Army Captain Anthony Smith suffered near fatal wounds while on duty in Iraq. Stationed near Baghdad with his unit, the Arkansas National Guard, Smith was hit by a two-metre-long rocket-propelled grenade. The missile lodged in his right hip and exploded, blowing off his right arm, ripping open his abdomen and destroying a kidney, shredding his intestines, and shattering his femur and right hip. The heat from the explosion burnt his retinas, and his dog tags were melted into his chest. As Smith staggered to his feet, he was shot four times by insurgents. Medical help reached him within minutes, but only in time to declare him dead, 'Killed in Action'. It was only as he was being zipped into a body bag that an observant soldier noticed an air bubble in Smith's neck, and realised he was still alive. Smith was rushed to a medical facility, where he began a long and painful path to recovery.[1]

Without a doubt, had Anthony Smith sustained such severe wounds in an earlier conflict he would not have survived. Advances in medical science and the treatment of war wounds have made it possible, even commonplace, for soldiers as badly wounded as Smith to be revived, treated and returned to their families. Doctors treating those with war wounds face new challenges, such as how to give the survivors a good quality of life and the ability to live as normally as possible. But the ability to save those who sustain such horrendous wounds in war is nevertheless remarkable, given that less than a century ago the prospect would have been unthinkable.

It is only in the last 90 or so years of modern warfare that great strides have been made in the treatment of war wounds. At first glance, war and medicine seem contradictory: the aim of war is to kill, while medicine, and the professionals who practise it, strive to heal. But the contradiction is only apparent: after all, nations involved in war need fit and healthy soldiers to maintain fighting capability, and the means to repair the effects of war in order to return men to action as quickly as possible. Little wonder then that twentieth-century wars have done so much to accelerate both major and minor medical advances, with many of the discoveries later translated into civilian practice. Before the First World War, in conflicts such as the American Civil War and the Boer War, many more soldiers died from illness than from war wounds. Of the 22,000 British troops who died during the Boer War, two-thirds were victims of infectious disease: typhoid, for example, was a greater killer than any armed opponent.[2] That situation changed after 1914, and the onset of the world's first modern industrial war.

Military historians of the First World War have frequently commented on the way military leaders struggled to adapt to fighting this new kind of warfare. Medical historians, too, have noted how the medical profession also struggled to cope with its effects: while 'a new, more brutal way of waging war was to cause confusion and uncertainty … out of the wreckage came innovations that changed the very practice of medicine'.[3] Some of the major innovations of this era are now commonplace. The practice of triage, or sorting casualties by the severity of their wounds, was first practised by the French during the war, then adopted by other nations. Triage is now standard practice in all emergency medicine. The French also began the practice of debridement, the surgical removal of foreign objects and dead or damaged tissue from a wound, in order to promote proper healing and prevent infection. After debriding a wound, doctors would use what became known as the Carrel–Dakin method of cleansing wounds, using a sodium hypochlorite solution, which resulted in far fewer amputations. As these practices became more commonplace in casualty clearing stations and field hospitals, the number of soldiers dying from wounds and disease began to decline.

Other major medical advances during this war included blood transfusions, the understanding and treatment of shell shock, reconstructive and plastic surgery, the diagnostic use of x-ray machines, maxillofacial and oral surgery, physical therapy and rehabilitation.[4] The challenges of dealing with the First World War's devastating effects on soldiers' minds and bodies were many, but on the whole the medical profession rose to the challenge, developing methods which they then took with them into civilian life before the world's next global conflict encouraged yet another spurt of development.

Some of the greatest medical advances of the Second World War involved new kinds of drugs used either to prevent or to treat infection. The greatest revolution in infection control came with the widespread use of penicillin, which entered large-scale military distribution in 1944. Penicillin proved to be extremely effective against a wide spectrum of infections and by the end of the war its use had largely eradicated the problem of wound infection. It also made significant inroads into the perennial problem of venereal disease among fighting forces. Other new drugs proved particularly effective for soldiers fighting in the tropics. The Germans developed a synthetic quinine for malaria, called Atabrine, which was soon put into mass production and became the standard anti-malarial drug of the war. Another significant development was the use of plasma and whole blood to maintain blood pressure and to counter the effects of shock in wounded soldiers.

Not all medical advances during the Second World War were attained ethically. The Germans and Japanese conducted many medical experiments on prisoners of war, including testing the effects of frostbite, disease control, and different surgical techniques. But much of the knowledge from such experimentation was gained by force and caused pain, humiliation and even death for the victims. After the war, doctors faced the dilemma of whether it was ever justifiable to use the knowledge gained under such conditions to benefit their patients. Some argued that since the data existed –

however unethically it might have been obtained – it was valid to use it, while others doubted whether any use of such tainted data could ever be justified.[5] In the event, many of these test results have been used in medical research since the war, sometimes with the blessing of the victims, who wanted their pain and suffering to be used for the good of others.

The Korean War brought a different sort of innovation to the advanced medical treatment of soldiers. The greatest development of that war was undoubtedly the mobile army surgical hospital (MASH), a portable medical facility that grew out of the field hospitals of the Second World War, and was developed further by the United States after 1945. The MASH facilities were ideally suited to the rugged terrain and poor roads and railways in Korea. They allowed surgical skill to be transported close to the front line. The use of aeromedical evacuation in combination with the MASH in Korea was another innovation. It began in 1950 when the US Army asked its air force to use helicopters to transport the seriously wounded from front-line clearing stations to MASH facilities. This was a revolutionary approach to the medical evacuation of soldiers, and it saved thousands of lives. Evacuation by helicopter in Korea was largely responsible for achieving a 2.4 per cent mortality rate for allied soldiers, the lowest rate for wounded in any war to that time.

Aeromedical evacuation was refined by American and Australian forces during the Vietnam War. Called casualty evacuation, or 'dust-off', more efficient and faster aircraft carrying up to ten patients could deliver their human cargo to world-class hospital facilities in minimal time. In contrast to the First World War when it could take days for a soldier to get proper surgery, a soldier in Vietnam could potentially be on the surgeon's table within 20 minutes of being wounded. The hospital mortality rate for Vietnam was 2.6 per cent.[6]

Preventative programs were used more in Vietnam than in any previous conflict, largely in an attempt to combat the conditions of jungle warfare, such as skin diseases and malaria, and to reduce absenteeism resulting from venereal disease. These programs met with mixed success, but improvements were made in dealing with burns associated with crashed aircraft, exposure to napalm and mishandling of flamethrowers. The drug Sulfamyalon and fluid resuscitation were both developed for use on burns, resulting in a 50 per cent reduction in mortality compared with Korea.[7]

In the 30 years between the Vietnam War and the recent large-scale commitment of foreign troops to Iraq and Afghanistan, major medical advances have continued to be made. Modern medical techniques and medicines have resulted in a 90 per cent survival rate for soldiers wounded in these conflicts. Predominant in soldiers' medical conditions now are post-traumatic stress disorder (PTSD) and traumatic brain and spinal injuries,[8] complicated conditions that often require years of treatment. The US Army is rehabilitating wounded servicemen and women by using extreme sports to rebuild muscles and self-confidence, and treating PTSD with revolutionary techniques, allowing many of those affected to return quickly to the field.

New techniques are being tested on the battlefield as well, including bandages never seen before. Haemostatic dressings are impregnated with substances which stop bleeding, and seal and protect wounds.[9] In addition, a new American Armed Forces Institute of Regenerative Medicine, involving researchers at two dozen institutions, is embarking on research that aims to repair human bodies by helping to regenerate living tissue, rather than by relying on artificial parts.[10] Such research has significant implications for the civilian world. With more soldiers surviving war wounds, the medical world is now confronted with the long-term treatment of men and women who may have survived their wounds but now live with the painful and debilitating consequences.

Many of these medical advances and issues are the subject of the chapters in this volume, which has its origins in an international conference held at the Australian War Memorial, Canberra, in September 2009. The two-day event brought together eminent historians specialising in the medical and demographic consequences of warfare; medical practitioners and researchers in the field of military medicine; and former and serving medical officers, surgeons, nurses and veterans. The participants explored the impact of war, wounds and trauma through the historical record and through personal experiences. Their presentations were informative, wide-ranging, and at times extremely moving. Historians, veterans and doctors all gave their perspectives of wounds and treatment, and a wide variety of topics were covered: mine casualties; fear of wounds and acute trauma on the battlefield; shell shock; self-inflicted wounds and combat fatigue; facially disfigured soldiers; advances in surgery; and the rehabilitation of wounded veterans. Some papers dealt with more controversial aspects, such as the debate over the effects of 'Agent Orange' in Vietnam, and the problems of living with the effects of war wounds.

Jay Winter, from Yale University, presented the keynote address to the conference and his paper forms the opening chapter of this volume. His discussion on shell shock and the Great War poses three critical questions: did the Great War open a new era in the history of disability and of our understanding of who the disabled are? Did the treatment of those disabled by war-related wounds change from being a matter of charity to a matter of rights? And to what extent did the class of disability that was psychological injury take on a metaphorical character in some countries, but not others? Winter answers all of these queries with great insight and compassion. He reminds readers that more recent diagnoses of 'combat fatigue' and PTSD have their origin in shell shock, and that the way that condition was recognised, treated and regarded after the Great War has influenced subsequent generations of medical professionals.

In the following chapter Australian War Memorial historian Ashley Ekins explores a different aspect of the psychological wounds of the First World War. He describes those who were 'reluctant warriors', young men who had been trained to fight and kill but lacked the will to do so, at times resorting to self-inflicted wounds to escape duty. These ranged from minor injuries and poisoning to shooting, mutilation and, in extreme cases, suicide. This aspect of the war has often been downplayed or ignored, but Ekins writes with compassion of the men driven to such extreme actions, and of the doctors who were charged – sometimes unwillingly – with identifying and reporting them.

Because of the nature of trench warfare during the First World War, large numbers of soldiers suffered extensive and disfiguring facial wounds. In her chapter, PhD candidate Kerry Neale charts the advances made in maxillofacial and reconstructive surgery during the war, as surgeons struggled to give new lives, and faces, to the victims of these horrific wounds. The success of surgeons such as Harold Gillies and Henry Pickerill, both New Zealanders, is explored in the context of their work at Queen Mary's Hospital, Sidcup, in London.

Whether they were sent home early as a result of their wounds, or arrived home at the end of the war, most soldiers returning from the First World War had been changed in some way. Some bore the scars in obvious wounds or disease, while others bore invisible but equally damaging psychological scars. Historian Marina Larsson examines the postwar life of these men and their families in her chapter 'The home is always here for him'. Drawing on her book, *Shattered Anzacs: living with the scars of war*, Larsson examines the vital role of family caregivers, especially wives and mothers, in healing the nation's soldiers after the war. On returning home, many Australian soldiers who were physically or mentally damaged by war spent weeks and months in repatriation hospitals. Most were discharged into their family's care, often with only limited medical support available. Families struggled with the physical, emotional and financial burdens of looking after their loved ones, usually ignored by the Repatriation Department. Their efforts are not on the public record and often invisible, so Larsson's research is an important step in bringing the efforts of these caring relatives to light.

Two chapters in this volume deal with particular aspects of the Second World War: namely, the treatment of Nazi concentration camp inmates, during the war and afterwards. In his chapter, British scholar Paul Weindling addresses the difficult ethical issue of medical testing carried out on prisoners of war. He looks at the case of a group of female inmates of Ravensbrück concentration camp, who had their legs gashed and deliberately infected. As Weindling explains, the testing resulted from the assassination of Himmler's deputy, Reinhardt Heydrich, in 1942; the SS surgeon in charge attempted to determine whether Heydrich's life might have been saved with more effective infection control. The female victims of the testing, who called themselves 'Rabbits' in protest, did not submit quietly, instead turning their suffering into resistance.

The treatment and rehabilitation of concentration camp inmates after the war is the subject of the following chapter by historian Debbie Lackerstein. She looks at the liberation of Nazi camps in 1945 and gives a moving account of the medical challenges facing those who first entered the camps. They discovered the most horrific conditions, with tens of thousands of survivors, most starving and many half-deranged, living side-by-side with corpses. The liberators struggled to deal with the scale of the suffering, and with the lack of supplies and knowledge about how to deal with the conditions they encountered. Many victims were effectively 'killed with kindness' when given inappropriate food, while others simply could not be saved in time. Lackerstein is critical of the lack of Allied preparation for the conditions encountered, but praises the efforts of everyone who tried desperately to save as many people as they could. Her chapter is a moving tribute to the survivors and to the liberators who were faced with an urgent and unspeakably awful task.

The next chapter is devoted to describing a remarkable Australian veteran of the Korean War. The medical work of Dr Bryan Gandevia, a regimental medical officer serving with 3RAR in Korea, is described by his son, Simon Gandevia, using his father's medical publications and his personal papers. Bryan Gandevia described the harsh and debilitating conditions facing soldiers during the Korean winter, and his frustration at the lack of public interest in the experiences of Australian soldiers during this 'forgotten war'. The author also details his father's great interest in and promotion of military-medical history, particularly displayed during his long tenure as a member of the Australian War Memorial council.[11]

The Vietnam War casts a long shadow over the veterans of that conflict, and various aspects of the war were the subject of several papers presented at the *War Wounds* conference. Despite greatly improved survival rates for those who were wounded or became ill during their service, the Vietnam War presented medical professionals with new challenges. David Bradford's chapter chronicles his experiences as a 'gunner's doctor' with 4th Field Regiment, Royal Australian Artillery. He discusses the perennial problem of venereal disease and how it was tackled in Vietnam. In part, this meant trying to instil caution in young soldiers who were living in constant danger and wanted to let off steam in the brothels of Vung Tau, but, more practically, it involved the widespread distribution of condoms. Bradford also describes the problems excessive drinking caused for morale and discipline among the troops.

The issue of compensation for Vietnam veterans is pursued in the next chapter by Elizabeth Stewart, which examines an almost unknown aspect of Australia's commitment to the Vietnam War and a group of veterans whose efforts have never been properly recognised. The story of Australia's 450 civilian medical personnel, who served in South Vietnam's provincial hospitals in surgical teams from 1964 to 1972, is one of dedication, hard work and a willingness by civilians to put their lives in danger in order to help the Vietnamese people. Often exposed to danger and war trauma, these highly experienced surgeons, nurses, anaesthetists, laboratory technicians and others achieved a great deal, often with very basic equipment and supplies. For many it was the experience of a lifetime, but for others it left a legacy of mental and physical illness. To date, successive governments have refused to recognise their status as war veterans, disallowing them access to the same medical compensation granted to other veterans.

Because it was an undeclared war, and deeply unpopular on the home front, the soldiers' participation in Vietnam was controversial and their homecoming was lukewarm at best, and traumatic for them at worst. Problems of alcoholism, drug addiction and PTSD were often hidden by veterans for many years, and then only dealt with after several decades. One of the most controversial medical issues after the war concerned the effects on veterans of herbicides, known widely as Agent Orange. Two authors in this volume, representing two sides of the debate, address the subject.

Vietnam veteran and campaigner Graham Walker charts the controversy that emerged in Australia during the 1980s. He discusses the findings of the Royal Commission set up to look at veterans' claims for compensation, examining the reasons why veterans were outraged at the Commissioner's findings. He then looks at the way the issue was recorded and assessed by medical historian Professor F.B. Smith in the Vietnam official history volume, *Medicine at War*. Walker takes issue with Smith's findings and details a number of points where he finds Smith's research at fault. He concludes his chapter with a call for the history of the Agent Orange issue in Australia to be rewritten, in order to include the results of more recent scientific research and an account of how those reports have affected the way the subject is now viewed by the Australian government.

The official historian of the Vietnam volumes, Peter Edwards, presents an alternative perspective. He examines events in the early 1990s, including reports produced in the United States and Australia, which are usually seen as a major turning-point in the long battle by veterans for compensation for illnesses caused by Agent Orange. Edwards also examines the relationship of these reports to Professor Smith's section of the official history, and disputes Walker's interpretation of Smith's work. His chapter takes into account the political climate in both countries over recent years, something which has greatly influenced the way in which the Agent Orange issue has unfolded. Finally, he suggests that by focusing solely on the effects of herbicide spraying, the veterans' lobby group has neglected the issue of legitimate compensation for a wider spectrum of medical conditions, including alcohol abuse, nicotine addiction and PTSD.

The volume concludes with three personal accounts: two by medics who treated soldiers in the field, one in Vietnam and one in Afghanistan, and the third by a soldier who received devastating wounds from a mine. Tony White was a regimental medical officer with 5RAR in Vietnam in 1966–67, and he writes movingly of his experiences treating mine casualties during Operation Renmark in

February 1967. Mine explosions in Vietnam caused havoc among Australian, American and South Vietnamese troops, and the operation White describes, in which two mines were detonated, was one of the earliest, and worst, examples of multiple mine casualties. White writes of his emotions when he first witnessed the scene, and of his regard for the men who were wounded and for those who assisted them.

Sharon Cooper, in her chapter on nursing in Afghanistan, displays the courage, humour and humility typical of so many medical professionals who have served in Australian armed forces. Severely injured during a helicopter crash while serving in East Timor, Cooper recovered sufficiently to lead a medical team to Afghanistan in 2008. She kept a detailed journal and recounts some of her entries in this chapter, to convey what it was like treating both civilian casualties of war and Australian servicemen and women wounded in battle. Cooper's account is a moving tribute to her own courage and that of her team mates who, like her, retain a strong belief in the worth of their work in such a dangerous part of the world.

In the concluding chapter, Vietnam veteran Graham Edwards movingly describes the experience of being wounded by a mine and his long and painful road of rehabilitation. Graham dealt with a repatriation system that was unable to cope with the physical and emotional needs of young men suffering devastating wounds and he writes with humour and pathos of his efforts to overcome his treatment and adjust to life without legs as best he could. His account of living life to the full in the face of such odds is testimony to the ability of the human spirit to prevail over adversity.

It is our hope that this collection of chapters, dealing as they do with such a wide variety of issues and conflicts, will help to bring to light some of the lesser-known aspects of the world's major twentieth-century conflicts. The interaction of medicine and war is not always well understood, nor is it given the attention it deserves, but we believe that this volume brings some of the most recent scholarship on this subject into the open. Doubtless it will promote much discussion and further research among its readers.

1

Shell shock and the lives of the Lost Generation

Jay Winter[1]

The wounds of war are with us still. The Russian poet Anna Akhmatova wrote these words in 1919:

> Why is this century worse than those that have gone before?
> In a stupor of sorrow and grief
> It located the blackest wound
> But somehow couldn't heal it.[2]

That wound was total war, and the violence embedded in it came to dominate the century that opened in 1914.

The wounds of the Great War lasted long after the Armistice of 1918. Some of the wounds of war did heal by themselves, by the intervention of time and only time; others healed by the intervention of people – doctors, nurses, health workers, and family members. The novelist Pat Barker said that women in countless families were and are the unsung healers of the wounded of war, and thereby came to join their ranks.[3]

It is necessary, I believe, to ask some difficult questions about our own subject position when we face those wounded in war. It is an essential moral act, I hold, to look at them. And yet that gaze is deeply problematic. If we turn away completely, we are hardly human; if we don't feel the impulse to turn away, we are not human at all. How do we look at the suffering of others? That is the question I, following Susan Sontag,[4] put to you in this chapter.

I ask this question in a particular context. It is that of the case of 'shell shock', a term invented during the Great War itself. I want to open the conversation about war wounds with this case, not because it is representative of the overall category, but because it shows the extent to which medical history and cultural history need to be braided together to guide us towards a fuller understanding of the long shadow of war.

Considering shell shock is useful in another way. It helps us see to what extent the Great War and the wounds inflicted during it shaped the century that has followed it. I want to address only three elements of this subject here. I do so in the form of three questions.

First, did the Great War open a new era in the history of disability, and of our understanding of who the disabled are? I believe the answer is yes. The Great War was the biggest industrial accident in history, but not only did it create more injuries than any that came before, it also transformed the framework of compensation and treatment for such injuries.[5] The history of orthopedic medicine and of rehabilitation medicine was transformed by the war; the history of other branches of medical care – neurology, psychiatry, surgery – was similarly transformed by war. Compensation for war-related injury required medical authorisation of the legitimacy of the claim. This brought bureaucrats and physicians into contact in ways and to a degree that had not happened before.

Secondly, did the treatment of disability for those suffering from war-related wounds change from being a matter of charity, of grace and favour, to being a matter of rights? I think the answer is more mixed, but by and large it is again yes. The Great War extended the right to medical care for a large population of people. After the war, that right became established practice in some countries and not in others. The notion that wounded men have a right to care was, to be sure, never uncontested, but it emerges everywhere, even in the United States, which – let us admit the shocking truth – has had socialised medicine for veterans for generations, a fact that still eludes a surprisingly large number of people.

For millions of men, the Great War led to the establishment of a right to care, over both the short- and long-term. And yet the differences between how combatant countries faced that fact were substantial. Here is where medical history and the history of veterans' movements and institutions come together. Let me give just one instance. In the period of the Great War in Britain, it was the injured soldier who had to prove that his injury was war-related; in France, for instance, it was the state which had to prove that the injury was not war-related. The burden of proof was on the individual in one country and on the state in another. I account for this distinction by referring to the differing stances adopted by veterans' associations in different countries, and to the relative power and influence of these associations. In Britain, the British Legion and other veterans' groups were essentially conservative in character, and embedded in the Protestant voluntary tradition of grace and favour. In France, veterans' associations were assertive and embedded in the Jacobin and Republican tradition of an armed citizenry.[6] I believe that all countries were arrayed somewhere between the two; as in the Australian case, there is a shifting landscape of entitlements, established by the determination of veterans' groups to press their case. It was a simple one. When it went to war, the state made a contract to look after the wounded, a contract which it was under an obligation not to break. After the war, governments and civil servants pushed back, to cut the costs of care and pensions, but they did so in different ways in different countries. The outcomes are complex, but it must be emphasised that whatever the level of reparation, it never fully compensates for the suffering and hardship the war wounded endured.

The third question I want to focus on concerns the traces of war-related disability in our language. To what extent did one class of disabilities – that of psychological injury or impairment – take on a metaphoric character in some countries and not in others, standing for the broader range of truncations and hardships that war leaves in its wake? In Britain, shell shock escaped from the medical realm into a metaphoric one; in France and Germany, however, where veterans' groups were stronger, shell shock – referred to by other terms – did not take on an iconic character. Only in Britain and in the Anglo-Saxon world did it do so.

Shell shock

The term 'shell shock' tells us a lot about the war. Most casualties were inflicted by artillery; the scale of the suffering and human costs of the war produced the shock. Here was a conflict which transformed the meaning of battle, of courage, of war itself. Here was a war in which the suffering did not end when the peace treaties were signed. It cast a shadow on men and their families for decades to come.

We are, therefore, in a space between military history and cultural history, a space given over to the study of the way contemporaries make sense of the violent world in which they live. The history of shell shock was part of that set of signifying practices, that transformation of language, brought about by the war.

The term 'shell shock' has a history we can trace. In 1915 the British psychiatrist Charles Myers introduced the term to describe a set of disabling injuries suffered by men at the front. The medical history of this term has been ably explored; less well documented is the way the appearance of thousands of men with psychological injuries has come to frame what we now term 'traumatic memory'. In common language, shell-shocked soldiers were the first carriers of post-traumatic stress disorder (PTSD) in the twentieth century.

It is important to note that the condition was not new; what was original was the diagnosis. There had been similar psychological wounds in the American civil war. Some were termed, again evocatively, 'soldiers' heart'. Later on, during and after the Second World War, 'combat fatigue' became the term of art. Then post-Vietnam doctors validated the current usage 'post-traumatic stress disorder'.

What happened was that a term initially limited in 1915 to those under artillery fire was extended to all those in combat 30 years later. After another 30-year interval, the term physicians and administrators used – PTSD – was not limited to men in uniform, but to many others afflicted by persecution, cruelty, and violence. Holocaust survivors are among them; so are the *hibakusha*, the survivors of Hiroshima and Nagasaki.

The cultural history of shell shock is, therefore, the story of its widening applicability, the creation, as it were, of a series of concentric circles of victims of war. Nowadays the term 'PTSD' extends to the domestic sphere. It has become universal. But it is important to recall the original setting of this category of psychological injury, the setting of the Great War. It took most of a century before the shame and stigma attached to mental illness were sufficiently reduced to enable societies to recognise the fact – the unalterably simple fact – that ordinary, healthy men break down in war. Through no fault of their own, and at the call of the state, they go into the shadows, shadows that stretch long into what we call the postwar world.

By the end of the twentieth century, the medical profession had recognised PTSD as a medical syndrome, with causes and treatment, and with legitimacy as a category of war-related injury. Even then, the veterans of Vietnam were not always well treated for these disorders; but because of their struggles today's soldiers have a better chance of receiving what is their right. The history of shell shock is in part the history of the struggle for veterans' rights and the search for natural justice.

In this context, we must therefore deal not only with politics and administration, but also with ordinary language, and with representations of war wounds embedded in it. These representations took many forms – medical, poetic, fictional, visual. We need to attend to them all to be able to comprehend why this phenomenon, arising in the 1914–18 conflict, has come to symbolise traumatic injury and traumatic memory in the century which followed the outbreak of the war.

First, what did the term mean to those who saw it during the Great War and after? Shell shock was not a new condition in 1914; rather it was a new diagnosis. Shell shock is a condition in which the link between an individual's memory and his identity is severed. A set of unassimilable images and experiences, arising from war service, either in combat or near it, radically disturbs the narrative, the life story, of individuals, the stories people tell themselves and others about their lives. Through such stories, we come to know who we are, or at least think we do.[7] Shell shock undermines that orientation, that point of reference, from which an individual's sense of self unfolds. His integrity, in the sense of his having an integral personality, one with a 'then' and a 'now' that flowed together, becomes uncertain because of what he has felt and seen and what he continues to feel and see. In many cases the visual imagination is central to this condition. Before the eyes of a shell-shocked man were images frequently of an uncanny, life-threatening, and terrifying kind, and they endure. Their meaning – that is, their location alongside other images and experiences – is unclear or bizarre. These visualised or felt traces of war experience can tend to live a life of their own, a life at times so vivid and powerful as to eclipse all others. They can paralyse; in extreme cases, they can kill. Suicide is the ultimate escape from them.

Fortunately, most of those who fought did not suffer from this condition, and most of those who did, were able to find a way to live with it or move beyond it. Their recovery was independent of many forms of medical care, since the pathways of causality in this area of neuro-psychology were unknown, and patterns of care were unsettled, contested and highly subjective. Many doctors made informed guesses, but the initial presumption of a purely organic cause of psychological disturbances had to be discarded over time. What would replace the initial, purely physical model of psychiatric illness was an open question; it remains open today. What is less elusive are the images of the men who suffered from the cluster of conditions we call shell shock.

Whatever the state of medical knowledge then, physicians still had a task to do. They had thousands of psychologically damaged soldiers to care for. The breakdown rate among Allied armies was not very different from the rate in the German and Austrian armies, but the recovery rate of such men was higher, in part because of the assembly-line treatment of these men. Recovery rates of 90 per cent were reported;[8] but surely these results simply meant that damaged men were declared healthy, then sent back to the front, where they broke down again. Reports of what we term shell shock were similar in all armies, though medical nomenclature and policy differed between and among them.[9] In every army, doctors did what they could, mostly through listening, caring, and counselling. In this way they played a real, though sometimes minor, role in the rehabilitation of these men. When discharged, shell-shocked men found much less sympathy from war pension officials, whose job primarily was to reduce the charge on the public purse rather than to meet the state's obligation to men suffering war-related injury.[10] Self-help, camaraderie, and family support were the most common paths to recovery for those not severely disabled.

Whatever the degree of disability they suffered, and however they were cared for, the presence in towns and villages, in cities and on the land, of thousands of shell-shocked men raises important issues for our understanding of the aftermath of war, and of the way the Great War configured different notions of memory at the time. Thinking about the term and the men whose lives it describes offers a framework within which to claim yet again that the survivors of the Great War constituted a 'generation of memory'. In this case the memories in question were disabling, disturbing, unassimilable.

Time and again after 1918, this form of troubled remembrance has been reconfigured in different ways, as combat fatigue or PTSD. But all discussions of the notion of traumatic memory sooner or later return to the scene of the crime, the site of combat in which the term 'shell shock' was invented and circulated.

Shell shock raised questions about the limits of discipline and duty during the Great War. Contemporaries had enormous trouble in comprehending a set of conditions that did not fit normative categories of behaviour under fire. At one pole stood rectitude, in the form of duty and stoical endurance; and at the other, deceit, in the form of feigned psychological injury. There were many good examples of both. But between the two was a vast array of men, whose condition barred them from duty through no fault of their own, and through no effort to deceive. The predicament of these men and those who treated them is at the heart of the history of shell shock.

Seeing embodied memory

One way to open this discussion of shell shock is to visualise it. Early in the war, army physicians began to handle cases of psychological breakdown, of paralysis and of disturbingly uncontrolled physical behaviour among men who had been in combat. From these cases, C.S. Myers and others coined the term 'shell shock', positing that some physical damage, such as concussion, arose from exposure to artillery fire and the like.[11] Though these physicians were later to distance themselves from this nomenclature, it stuck.[12] It is important to try to see the phenomenon with their eyes. What was it that these physicians saw? We know something about this question from training films for doctors made in the war. The disturbing character of these images, I believe, lay both in the body of the sufferer and in the gaze of the onlooker. Together they (and we) share embodied memory.[13] In almost every instance, the conversion of emotional states to physical ones is apparent. The involuntary movement of the jaw of a man who had bayoneted another locates the incident in his own body. His body is telling the story of what he had done. There are war stories too in the unsuccessful efforts of a man trying to stand up or the tremors of the man whose walking is not under control and bears a curious resemblance to Charlie Chaplin's trademark gait. We can simply ask where had their legs taken them? Their bodies bore the traces of combat. There is embodied memory too in the case of a man who responds to nothing other than the word 'bomb', which (when heard) sends him scurrying under the bed; and in the terrified response of a French soldier triggered by the sight of an officer's hat. These soldiers have internalised memory; it is inside them, and when touched, their bodies respond as if they were sprung coils.[14]

Here we can see and feel one kind of embodied memory. It is written on the men who fought, or inscribed in them in a way that is not subject to their direct or premeditated control. In all instances,

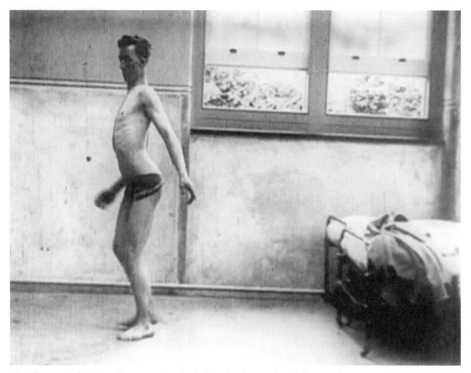

The 'hysterical' gait of a severely shell-shocked British soldier undergoing treatment at Netley Hospital in England in 1917. (Still photograph from motion picture, 'War Neuroses: Netley Hospital, 1917', courtesy of the Wellcome Library, 2042F.)

images and memories seem to live both embedded in these people and curiously detached from them; memory itself, or images of over-whelming events, appear to be free-floating powerful agents which somehow control the jaw of a man, or his leg, or all his movements.

In effect, these men's bodies perform something about their war experience. Shell shock is a theatre of memory out of control. The bodies of these soldiers hold traces of memory; they are speaking to us, though not in a way which we usually encounter. Here stories become flesh; physical movements occur without end or direction, or there is no movement at all.

If memories tell us who we are, then what did these powerful memory traces of combat tell these men about who they were? These images, feelings, and memories didn't fit; they could not be interpolated into a story of 'before and after'. They challenged and sometimes even fragmented identity, and one of the fragments overwhelmed all others. It is this kind of frozen moment that we see in these images;

a few gestures concentrate those events and the memories of them. Sometimes soldiers (with or without the aid of physicians) could specify what these memories were. It may have been an incident in combat; at other times, crucial events were more difficult to locate. But in all these cases, bodies seem to remember something; they engage in a kind of unwitting re-enactment that tended to defy both verbal expression and the urge to forget.[15]

I want to turn now to the second sense of embodied memory, that related to those who viewed these images, or saw these men or thousands like them. These films were made to train physicians as to what they should do with psychologically damaged soldiers. Most army doctors were at a loss as to how to help these men; Freud was similarly puzzled and uncertain.[16] We know that other physicians – the Austrian physician and future Nobel laureate, Julius Wagner-Jauregg, for instance – used electro-convulsive shock treatment to discourage malingering. In these films we see traces of the use of electricity to stimulate recalcitrant muscles to help do their job, and to help a man clearly struggling to walk again. No malingering here. We know that other physicians used electro-convulsive shock treatment in even more radical ways, though these celebrated cases were exceptional.[17] What were the lessons learned by the original viewers of these images, the medical men whose job it was to try to make them better? It is hard to say precisely; such evidence as we have indicates that these images were used to help separate the malingerer from the legitimate sufferer of shell shock. The movements of these men are not conjured up; the men can't repeat them on request, because they are automatic or uncontrolled. Charlie Chaplin may walk with an awkward gait, and make us feel he is about to fall, but everyone knows it is an act: he can start it or stop it at will. These men, however, are not acting. Wartime film footage was there to better enable physicians to tell who was really sick and who was simply trying it on. How to separate the two was a virtually impossible task, but visual evidence was there to help.

The therapeutic context was only one site where such images appeared. Other soldiers saw such men, and so did civilians, when the soldiers were sent back from casualty clearing stations to base hospitals or home, or when they returned to the front and broke down again, a far from uncommon occasion. These injured men were there, an integral part of the community of soldiers, not so much a nation as a brotherhood, the *'génération du feu'*, *'ceux de '14'*. And yet their illnesses were so odd, so frightening, that their presence was always a problem. The stigma of mental illness did not vanish just because it was registered in the service of one's country. To see such men was to encounter a side of war no one wanted to confront.

Shell-shocked men were not the only people hard to face in the postwar world. The *gueules cassées*, or disfigured men, were there too. So were the amputees and those with prosthetic arms and legs. Otto Dix painted them on street corners in Germany, or playing cards in a harsh satiric reconfiguration of Cézanne's *Les joueurs de carte (The card players)* of 1890–92.

My fundamental point is that these men challenged contemporary understandings of what war wounds were and of the lives of those who bore their traces. The images these men had in their minds did not fade when they left the field of battle. Conventional notions of masculinity or stoicism did not hold when men of unquestionable courage broke down under the weight of their memories. Those who saw these medical training films were viewing memories that had taken over the lives of the men who had them. These people were walking arguments against the view that demobilisation came to an end when the last serving soldier in a combat unit left the service. Mental illness – as much as physical disabilities – told another story, one that lingered.

There is another group of observers whose thinking on the meaning of shell shock we need to think about. What do we see when we gaze at these images? We see men who suffer; men like us. We see their embodied memory, and link it to what we think we know about war and its aftermath. How this happens is a complicated and lengthy story, but my guess is that for several generations, in some countries and not in others, such images have been fundamental in establishing what Samuel Hynes calls a 'war-in-the-head',[18] the mental furniture we all have about war and what it does to people. It challenges our understanding of what war is, and indeed our understanding of what memory is.

It is important to note the culturally differentiated nature of this argument. In Britain (but not to the same degree or in the same way in France or Germany) as a result of stories, poems, and especially images, successive generations have inherited a set of icons or metaphors about the war. Shell shock is one such metaphor. Metaphors are always open to interpretation. But they have truths in them to which their survival attests. One of them is that battle does not end when the firing stops; it goes on in the minds of many of those who returned intact, or apparently unscathed, and in the suffering of those whose memories are embodied, enacted, repeated, performed.

How do we look at these images? Are we voyeurs? Should we be ashamed to look on them? I think not, because looking at war, really looking at it, requires us to see, to recognise, to acknowledge, what it does to the bodies and minds of the men who fight. Shell shock, in sum, is a condition that happens when the link is severed between memory and identity. When memories cannot be interpolated into the stories we tell ourselves about who we are. That story is with us still.

Conclusion: the legacy of shell shock

One way in which to frame the history of shell shock is to examine the phenomenon as a kind of syntax of war, an ordering of stories and events elaborated by men who served. In this narrative, some men never demobilised; they were frozen in time, not out of choice, but out of injury, internal injury known only to them. The suffering of these men, so resistant to medical treatment, was both a reminder and a reproach. It disrupted heroic narratives of the war, and challenged conventional interpretations of its meaning. It made everyone – patriots as well as ordinary onlookers – uncomfortable. Shell shock placed alongside one line of temporality, in which there was ante-bellum and post-bellum, another sense of time, what some scholars call 'traumatic time'.[19] It is circular or fixed rather than linear. Here the clock doesn't move in a familiar way; at times its hands are set at a particular moment in wartime, a moment which may fade away, or may return, unintentionally triggered by a seemingly innocuous set of circumstances. When that happens, a past identity hijacks or obliterates present identity; and the war resumes again.

This kind of arrested demobilisation is embedded in 'traumatic memory', and much of the way we understand the concept today, and its relevance to the victims of current conflicts, rests on a reading of this aspect of the history of the Great War.[20] That this phenomenon is only part of the legacy of the war needs emphasis. The subject of 'traumatic memory' is of fundamental importance, but it must not replicate its referent and eclipse other narratives of war. The years after the Armistice were a time when competing and contradictory narratives were elaborated, at times by different people, at times by the same person, at different stages of his or her life. Duty, deceit, and disturbance were there in abundance. The messy, unstable, unsettled character of demobilisation derives from this war of narratives, a war that has gone on and on, and still can be heard now, nearly a century after the Great War began. Shell shock is at the heart of narratives of imprisoned memories, of broken identities and of identities restored. By bequeathing to us these terms and images of war wounds, the survivors of the Great War fashioned themselves as central figures in the first, though by no means the last, generation that has had to confront the terrible violence of the twentieth century and beyond.

'Chewing cordite': self-inflicted wounds among soldiers of the Great War

Ashley Ekins

Soldiers of the Great War inhabited a world of wounds and mutilation. The immense casualty rates in that first mass, industrialised war of the 20th century exposed men to the constant sight, sound, smell and the seemingly random risk of death and maiming. Something of the monstrous scale of the conflict is conveyed in the raw statistics of death and wounds within the armies of 1914–18. On the Western Front, the British army incurred almost 2.7 million battle casualties, one-quarter of them killed, and over half of all British soldiers who served suffered some kind of wound in battle. In the French army on the Western Front the figures were even higher: there were almost 4 million battle casualties among the 6.3 million troops mobilised, amounting to 62 per cent of all men in uniform. In the Australian force, of some 331,000 who embarked for service overseas, almost 65 per cent became casualties: approximately 215,000 men, of whom 60,000 died on active service.[1]

Most soldiers became inured to the grim experiences they

repeatedly faced. But in every war theatre and every national army, the prolonged strain of static trench warfare and sustained artillery bombardment eroded troops' morale and undermined their discipline and fighting spirit. This was particularly the case in the worst periods on Gallipoli and the Western Front: for Australian soldiers, most notably during the winter at Flers at the conclusion of the Somme offensive of 1916, in the closing phases of the Third Ypres offensive in late 1917, and during the intense fighting of the German spring offensive in April 1918. In such periods, a significant minority succumbed to the trauma of shell shock. The number of shell-shock cases in the British Army increased four-fold during the battle of the Somme, from 3951 cases in the first six months of 1916 to 16,138 in the last six months of the year, a number equivalent to an entire division.[2]

Some soldiers took matters into their own hands and actively sought escape through various means to avoid military duty and danger. The methods men employed for malingering and shirking – 'swinging the lead' in the soldiers' slang of the period – were staggering in their variety and inventiveness, particularly at the less serious end of the scale when attempting to avoid military parades, fatigues and other duties. Soldiers feigned a wide range of diseases and conditions, including shell shock, appendicitis, lumbago, deafness, blindness, insanity and epileptic fits, sometimes cutting their gums and placing soap in their mouths to create frothing. They took drugs to simulate respiratory and circulatory system disorders; they ingested picric acid to imitate jaundice; they put irritants in their eyes to simulate conjunctivitis; they deliberately infected slight injuries; and they injected petrol, paraffin or turpentine into knee joints to induce synovitis and abscesses.[3]

Some even deliberately sought to acquire venereal diseases, despite the severe consequences, both physical and military. Punishments included stoppages of pay and the shame of incarceration in military 'dermatological hospitals', such as the Australian establishment at Bulford, England, or that at Langwarrin Camp in Victoria, which were in many respects more akin to military prisons.

It was the responsibility of army doctors, or regimental medical officers (RMOs), to detect malingerers and expose them in order to maintain discipline in units and to keep the sick lists low. While sustaining soldiers' health and morale, doctors were expected to identify and report suspected offenders. Many developed specialist skills in this 'detective' work. The practice often blurred the boundaries between treatment and coercion as regimental doctors became agents of military justice, often unwillingly.[4]

A British doctor who served with the Fourth and Fifth Armies in France told the War Office enquiry into shell shock in 1922 that he found it 'an extremely difficult and distasteful task' to give evidence in courts martial regarding the mental and medical state of soldiers charged with serious cases of malingering and desertion. In almost all cases, he gave evidence in favour of the men charged, believing they were not responsible for their actions under the stresses of combat and shell fire.[5]

There were also men like Captain J.C. Dunn of the 2nd Battalion, Royal Welch Fusiliers, who typified the finest type of regimental medical officer. Dunn was a 'hard-bitten man' according to one famous officer of the battalion, author and poet Robert Graves, and had no sympathy for malingerers and shirkers. He was a professional soldier as well as a doctor. On one occasion at Polygon Wood during the Third Battle of Ypres in 1917, Dunn even armed himself with a rifle, bayonet and bandolier of ammunition and unofficially took command of a mixed group of British and Australian troops, firmly leading them in repelling a German counter-attack.[6]

Dunn believed the 'first duty of a battalion medical officer in War is to discourage the evasion of duty'. Among the rank and file, 'neither "Old Sweats" nor young conscripts could attempt to "swing the lead" with Dunn'. He knew all the dodges soldiers might try, including the ploy of chewing a stick of cordite, extracted from a .303 cartridge, to induce a high temperature and irregular heartbeat. Invariably, 'M&D', medicine and duty, was his standard response to 'scrimshankers' at morning sick parades. But Dunn was also 'sensitive to the effects of stress on the infantry . . . [and] attempted to give aid and comfort to those who were temporarily unable to stand the strain'.[7] A good RMO, noted another doctor, Charles Wilson of the 1st Battalion,

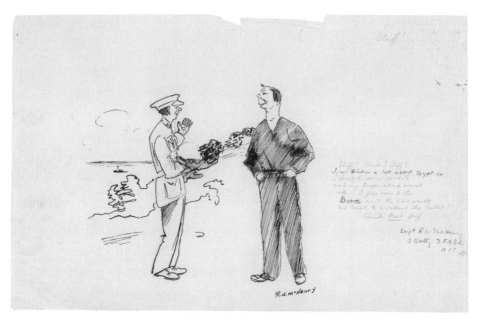

An Australian soldier's cartoon rejected for publication in *The Anzac Book*, Gallipoli, November 1915. 'I chewed some cordite,' says one soldier, 'and my temperature went up. I goes over to the Doc and the cow sends me back to swallow the bullet. Ain't *that* stiff?' (AWM RC09647, original art work in MSS1316/3/4, box 2.)

Royal Fusiliers, watched his men closely for 'signs of wear and tear, [so] that a man might be rested before he was broken'. Men 'wore out like clothes', he observed, and every man, no matter how brave, would eventually reach his limit.[8]

Soldiers could often find humour in unlikely situations, even the morning sick parade. In November 1915 an Australian soldier submitted his comic sketch as a contribution for *The Anzac Book*, a collection of soldiers' art and writing compiled on Gallipoli by Australian official war correspondent Charles Bean as a diversion for the troops during the approaching winter. The sketch depicted an Australian soldier complaining that his attempt at malingering had been detected by a sceptical doctor, no doubt an experienced officer like Dunn:

> "Stiff? Ain't I stiff?", he says. "I was thinkin' a lot about Egypt so I chewed some cordite and my temperature went up. I goes over to the Doc and the cow sends me back to swallow the bullet. Ain't *that* stiff?"[9]

Bean rejected the cartoon for the publication perhaps because of its subversive tone and because it did not accord with the idealised image of the Anzac digger that he wanted to present.

Army doctors also issued prescription compounds containing tincture of iron perchloride which stained the mouth, so that soldiers who were deliberately trying to prolong illness by not taking their medication could be discovered. Another Australian soldier-artist depicted a malingering digger's attempt to blame the doctors for his feigned 'condition':

> Doctor (doubting, hands on hips): "What's wrong with you?"
>
> Digger: "Well if y'arst me ter diagonise meself, I'd say it wus an over-dose of tin'ture of iron in block form wot settled on me stummick."[10]

Despite the humorous treatment, malingering was an ever-present reality and senior commanders recognised its potentially corrosive effects on discipline, particularly in Australian units. Throughout the war, Australian troops were generally regarded as the most refractory element in the British army.[11] In August 1918 the Adjutant General reported that the number of Australian soldiers committed to military prisons in the previous six months almost equalled the total for the remainder of the British armies in France, and they gave 'more trouble in the prisons than all the other troops put together'. Australian soldiers in military prisons showed considerable ingenuity in the methods they used to render themselves unfit for front line service. According to the Adjutant General:

> They have been known to maim themselves by putting pieces of wire into their knees, and injecting petrol, which makes the joint stiff, while cases of gonorrheal opthalmia, which are considered to be self-inflicted, are of frequent occurrence, and special precautions have to be taken accordingly in the prison hospitals.[12]

Aside from those in prisons, significant numbers of soldiers in all national armies resorted to extreme measures to avoid service in the front line and going into battle. They disabled themselves with self-inflicted wounds caused by shooting and various forms of self-mutilation; in extreme cases, some even chose suicide. The official histories were generally silent about such incidents or diminished their significance.

Some historians have argued that the Australian official historian Charles Bean downplayed the incidence of indiscipline, particularly the frequency of self-inflicted wounds, malingering and even occurrences of cowardice, combat refusals and retreating in panic from the enemy.[13] But Bean's volumes contain more references to indiscipline than any comparable official history of the Great War. Perhaps it is the brevity and the sometimes ambiguous nature of most of these references, together with Bean's failure to quantify or estimate the numbers of men involved, that encouraged this later criticism. Bean could be relatively frank and forthright in his personal diaries. On Gallipoli, he noted:

> the nonsense [in the popular press] about wounded soldiers wanting to get back from hospital to the front. . . everyone here knows that it is not one soldier in fifty that wants to go back to the front. They dread it. Not very many will actually shoot their fingers off to escape from the front, but even this is not uncommon even among Australians and it is probably less common with them than with most.[14]

But even if Bean had been inclined to expand on these issues in his official history, the quantified information he would have needed was not readily available to him or any other researcher. Colonel A.G. Butler, author of the medical volumes of the Australian official history, dealt with the subject of discipline and morale in greater detail than Bean and discussed such discipline-related medical problems as self-inflicted wounds and malingering with considerable frankness.[15] Butler also recorded, in passing, the total numbers of the most frequent offences dealt with by courts martial in the combined British forces during the war; but he noted his frustration that 'corresponding figures relating to the A.I.F. alone cannot be obtained', because 'the main records of the Provost Marshal's Department in Australia were destroyed after the war and the official conviction forms have not been consolidated'. Butler added that statistics for 'malingering' in the Australian force were 'practically non-existent, owing to the absence of any exact study of the experiences in the War of the Department of the Judge Advocate General'.[16]

The problem of precise measurement was compounded by the destruction of the medical records. Charles Bean recorded in his diary on 14 December 1915 that during the preparations for the evacuation from Gallipoli, 'The orderly of the 1st Divl [Divisional] Medical Branch burnt by mistake all their records this morning!'[17] There was a more serious loss of invaluable medical records when in 1923 the British Office of Works in London destroyed all the Australian Imperial Force (AIF) soldiers' medical record cards. These clinical and statistical records were an irreplaceable loss to the medical, military and social history of Australia (and also of Canada whose records were similarly destroyed). Butler and his small team, over many years and 'by colossal labour', completed the task of reconstituting and compiling a mass of statistical information on casualties and disease from hospital Admission and Discharge books.[18] But the task of consolidating the medical records in soldiers' service records, still awaits an energetic and inspired research student, or perhaps a team. In the absence of such data, most published accounts remain based largely on anecdotal and impressionistic evidence.

The number of recorded charges for self-inflicted wounding undoubtedly underestimated the full extent of this problem on Gallipoli. Many wounds were not identified as self-inflicted and were treated as ordinary wounds sustained in action. Butler noted the difficulties faced by the military authorities in controlling the 'repeated short epidemics of self-inflicted wounds' on Gallipoli.[19]

From the early months of the war, 'Blighty' wounds, which offered escape from the front line were welcomed. As one long-serving

British soldier recalled during the First Battle of Ypres in October 1914, 'even at this time we used to reckon that anyone who got a clean wound through the leg or arm was an extremely fortunate man'.[20] Those who attempted to inflict a convincing wound themselves were not always so lucky. Captain Dunn recorded in late November, after the first heavy snow and frost of a freezing winter:

> A man shot himself through the arm, 'probably on purpose'. He was not the first of whom that is said, or by any means the last. This man took ingenious precautions to conceal the evidence of a point-blank shot. He died of haemorrhage.[21]

Occasionally soldiers assisted others in either maiming themselves or in escaping detection after shooting themselves. An Australian soldier of the field ambulance recorded that he treated one man's self-inflicted gunshot wound by covering the gunpowder burn marks with repeated iodine applications and warned him to keep applying the iodine until the wound blistered to remove the burnt skin: 'Poor beggar had been a good soldier prior to this and was not really responsible for his nerve collapse. Am glad to say he escaped detection and subsequently made good. S.I. wounds are very rare indeed.'[22]

As the war dragged on, the prolonged ordeal of 'the human grindstone' of war on the Western Front began to wear down men's resistance and will to fight. As one historian observed:

> There were few men who did not dream of receiving a wound that, though not bad enough to kill, ensured one's being invalided out of the army. Talk in the trenches came back again and again to the legendary 'blighty one' or 'jammy one', and the chances of being crippled or disfigured were gladly reckoned with as long as it meant escape from the line. For the French such a wound was known as *une 'bonne' blessure*.[23]

After enduring months of the monotonous ordeal of Gallipoli and that campaign's constant dangers, disease and death, many Australian soldiers saw a 'holiday wound' as 'the only passport to genuine rest', observed historian Bill Gammage. As winter approached, few wounded men were anxious to return to the besieged beachhead at Anzac Cove. Some soldiers lasted only a few days, like one 'new arrival' mentioned in an officer's diary, who 'deliberately shot off his foot'.[24]

How widespread was the resort to self-maiming? Some authorities, such as Major General Sir Wyndam Childs, Deputy Adjutant General, who was well placed to know the true extent of the problem, claimed it was 'a very prevalent crime'.[25] But the actual *recorded* frequency is low. This apparent paradox has led to some contrary conclusions among historians. Richard Holmes maintains that in formations for which there are extant records, the number of convictions for self-inflicted wounds appears to have remained relatively low.[26] Niall Ferguson argues that 'immediate, certain, self-inflicted pain rarely seems preferable to future and possibly avoidable pain inflicted by others' and consequently, 'the numbers of SIWs [self-inflicted wounds] and suicides was never very high'.[27] John Keegan, on the other hand, has stated that the advances in medical treatment during the Great War made such an option more reasonable to men under stress and fearful of the consequences. Keegan estimated that accidental wounds comprised 'at least five per cent of all woundings between 1914 and 1918', providing a welcome passport to excuse men from the obligation to 'jump the bags' and go into action.[28] Reported low numbers may perhaps be due to the difficulties involved in distinguishing between accidental wounds and those inflicted willingly as a means of escape from the battle front.

A clearer picture emerges from a detailed study of the surviving records. Canadian scholar James Brent Wilson concluded that in the British Army on the Western Front, self-inflicted wounds were much more prevalent than generally believed. The incidence of cases rose between August 1916 and October 1918 during 'the period of the big battles, which suggests that, like shell shock, it was linked to the stress of prolonged fighting.' By mid October 1916 during the battle of the Somme, the offence became widespread. The British 6th Division reported *37* soldiers admitted to hospital suffering self-inflicted wounds over just four days in early November; the commander of the 5th Division appealed to soldiers to co-operate in detecting 'malingerers' by reporting such cases, a largely ineffectual measure since most men were reluctant to inform on their comrades.[29]

Overall, the total numbers both of cases admitted to hospitals and of recorded convictions remained relatively low. British soldiers were charged by courts martial with 3904 cases of self-inflicted wounds, just over one per cent of the total number of 343,153 courts martial charges.[30] The official Australian figure of 700 medically reported cases on the Western Front is believed to considerably underestimate the actual number.[31] Despite the evidence from Butler's laboriously reconstituted medical records of the AIF it is clear that an unknown number simply went unreported.[32]

How large was this number? This author's own study of the AIF disciplinary records reveals that a total of 467 courts martial of Australian soldiers involved charges for self-inflicted wounds (just 1.27 per cent of the total).[33] But, based on the evidence from other sources, these reported and charged cases would appear to represent just a small proportion of a substantial unrecorded total. The AIF findings derive mainly from the examination of two sources: the disciplinary records which provide some more concrete evidence about the nature and circumstances of self-inflicted wounds; and the official reports, orders and instructions issued by unit and formation headquarters in the field, which indicate obliquely the scale of the problem through commanders' concerns about the incidence of self-inflicted wounds.

Examination of disciplinary cases from two main theatres, Gallipoli and the Western Front, provides some illuminating insights.

Gallipoli

From the outset, medical arrangements on Gallipoli were primitive and inadequate. There were some improvements as the campaign progressed but the harsh terrain and climate, the isolation of the peninsula, and the absence of any respite from the continual enemy fire and heavy fatigues, all took their toll of soldiers' morale. Within months it became clear to most men that their attempt to seize the

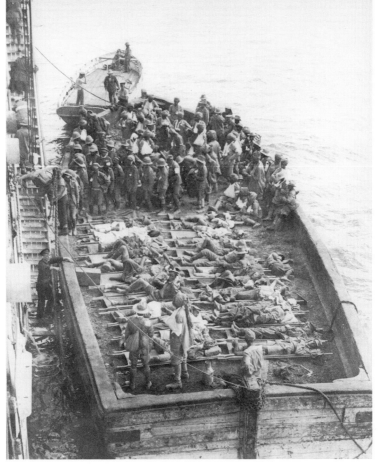

A barge transporting walking wounded soldiers and stretcher cases from Anzac Cove to the hospital ship *Gascon*. The notoriously inadequate medical arrangements during the Gallipoli campaign were later the subject of investigation during the Dardanelles Royal Commission. (AWM A02740)

Gallipoli peninsula had stalled and that there was no alternative to the prolonged stalemate of static trench warfare from which their only escape might be by death or wounds.

As a regimental medical officer on Gallipoli, Butler experienced at first hand the 'repeated short epidemics of self-inflicted wounds' he later described in his official history.[34] From less than one month after the landing, special instructions had to be issued regularly by units, warning of the problem: they cautioned that the wounded men in these cases of 'suspected or apparent self injury' were to be arrested and formally charged, and were not to be evacuated sick from the peninsula to hospitals. If men had to be evacuated they were not to be sent further than the main British base at Mudros Harbour on Lemnos island.[35]

With the onset of summer heat, sickness became endemic among soldiers worn down by unceasing manual labour under enemy fire, poor food and inadequate sanitation where plagues of flies were attracted to unburied dead bodies in no man's land and the open latrines. The result was a number of debilitating diseases including chronic diarrhoea and dysentery. In August a regimental medical officer reported: 'Men who were just skin and bone; hands, arms, and legs covered with septic sores; ill with dysentery; had to work in the trenches on bully-beef, bacon and biscuits.' One month later, a clinical examination of the health of Australian troops in the Anzac area found that 50 per cent of them had heart disorders, almost 80 per cent were emaciated, anaemic and suffering from intermittent diarrhoea, and over 60 per cent had skin ulcers.[36]

A British doctor who examined soldiers evacuated from Gallipoli to the island of Lemnos in November and December 1915 during the final phase of the campaign, told the War Office shell-shock enquiry:

> practically every man coming out of the Peninsula was neurasthenic, whether he was supposed to be fit or not. Very few could hold their hands out without shaking, and they were all in a condition of profound neurasthenia. The vast majority of the men at that time were suffering from dysentery, and a great number of them had jaundice as well.[37]

He believed the general debilitation of the soldiers was due to the combined effects of disease and the strain of being under constant shell fire. The result was:

> an extreme degree of physical weakness, and very few men could carry their packs on the march. They arrived at Lemnos after the evacuation, and their power of marching had entirely disappeared. They had to rest every hundred yards or so. It was a condition of absolute exhaustion.[38]

Soldiers' morale and fighting spirit declined with their wasting physical condition. Twenty cases of self-inflicted wounds were reported in the single month of October within the 2nd Australian Division on Gallipoli.[39] By November, up to six men at any time were in the field ambulance dressing stations with self-inflicted wounds, generally gunshot wounds to the left hand.[40] Courts martial awarded increasingly severe punishments to those charged with the offence. The following case examples from an analysis of the Australian disciplinary records convey something of the harsh realities.[41]

On 6 November 1915 in the front line trenches at Quinn's Post on Gallipoli a private of the 17th Battalion blew off the index finger of his right hand with his rifle. He was charged with 'wilfully maiming himself with intent thereby to render himself unfit for service'. The soldier claimed his rifle discharged accidentally when he picked it up to fire from a post. He was sentenced to 60 days' Field Punishment No. 2, a common sentence involving stoppages of pay and extra fatigues and duties. Two days later, on 8 November in Leane's Trench, a private of the 1st Battalion shot himself in the palm of his left hand. He claimed the injury was caused by an accidental discharge while cleaning his rifle. He was sentenced to 6 months' imprisonment with hard labour, later commuted to 3 months' Field Punishment No. 1, similar to Field Punishment No. 2 but also requiring the soldier to be tied up to a fixed object for up to two hours each day.[42] The following week, on 16 November near the support trenches at Lone Pine, a private of the 23rd Battalion shot himself in the leg while at the latrines. The court martial sentenced him to 6 months' imprisonment with hard labour, with no remission or suspension permitted.

Although the total number of cases was comparatively small, the incidence of the charge of self-inflicted wounding on Gallipoli was three times greater than the incidence of this charge within the AIF overall throughout the war.[43] Moreover, the number of charges for self-inflicted wounding undoubtedly underestimates the full extent of this problem on Gallipoli. Many wounds were not identified as self-inflicted and were treated either as ordinary wounds sustained in action or regarded as accidental. Nevertheless, commanders continued to regard the numbers of such cases as a revealing index of the state of morale and fighting efficiency within their units, together with the frequency of casualty evacuations for shell shock, and courts martial for related offences such as absence, desertion and disobedience.[44]

The Western Front

The intensity of large-scale warfare on the Western Front put increased pressure on soldiers and pushed many beyond their limits of resilience. The performance of the first Indian formations to join the British Army in France showed how extreme the phenomenon of self-inflicted wounds might become – particularly when the morale of troops unaccustomed to the Western Front was worn down by exposure to trench warfare, to the wet and cold weather, and the relentless casualties from enemy artillery.

After initially displaying good fighting qualities, large numbers of Indian soldiers of the Lahore and Meerut Divisions apparently began shooting themselves in the left hand in order to escape the front line. There was a copy-cat character to the practice. In a single two-week period in October and November 1914, 57 per cent of the 1848 Indian soldiers admitted to hospital were suffering hand wounds believed to be self-inflicted.[45] Over the ensuing winter, five Indian soldiers were executed for cowardice and the incidence of hand wounds reportedly dropped sharply.[46] But the Indian divisions were now considered unreliable for war on the Western Front. By November 1915 they were withdrawn from France and despatched to Mesopotamia. British senior commanders believed the problems stemmed from a shortage of British officers in the divisions and the inability of Indian troops to cope with the cold weather; these explanations actually ignored systemic inequities within the Indian Corps that affected the troops' morale.[47]

Nevertheless, the wearing effects of harsh weather and the constant strain of modern 'industrial' war on soldiers on the Western Front could not be discounted. The regimental medical officer, Captain Dunn, recorded his reflections in April 1917 on the deterioration of his own physical state and morale while living in reserve trenches. Around him were the sights and sounds of continuous battle and the bodies of dead soldiers lying in front of the trenches while he struggled to obtain the basic human requirements of food, warmth and sleep: 'infantry soldiering in the battle-zone was an overwhelmingly physical experience', he noted drily.[48]

Soldiers of the New Zealand division also suffered from their sudden exposure to the intensity of warfare on the Western Front. From the time they entered the trenches in May 1916, there was a rapid increase in the numbers of men wounding themselves to escape the front line, despite warnings that the crime would be treated seriously by courts martial and that those found guilty would incur severe punishments. As in other forces, men who suffered gunshot wounds in suspicious circumstances, usually claiming accidental discharges, were invariably treated as if the wounds were self-inflicted.[49]

A.G. Butler believed that self-inflicted wounds were less common among Australian troops in France because the 'motive that caused this on Gallipoli was largely absent on the Western Front', presumably referring to the isolated conditions, absence of relief in rear areas and the constant exposure to enemy fire on Gallipoli that drove men to such desperate measures in an attempt to escape.[50] But the medical and disciplinary statistics tell a different story. Cases of self-maiming became prevalent among Australian soldiers again from July 1916 when they endured unprecedented heavy artillery bombardments on the Somme. There were 128 charges for self-inflicted wounds in 1916 (4.2 per cent of total charges, compared with 1.1 per cent in the British army); 33 cases occurred in August alone, the most gruelling month of combat intensity.[51]

During the battles on the Somme and at Verdun in 1916, and at Passchendaele in 1917, the utter misery of soldiers' conditions produced further 'epidemics' of self-inflicted wounds in all armies. The phenomenon undoubtedly reflected the state of battle exhaustion and declining morale among troops, but within Australian and British units at least, there was little attempt to record the extent of self-inflicted wounds except as a measure of indiscipline.

By the end of the Somme campaign in November 1916, the morale of Australian soldiers reached its lowest point: some groups of men avoided tours in the trenches by malingering; and individuals

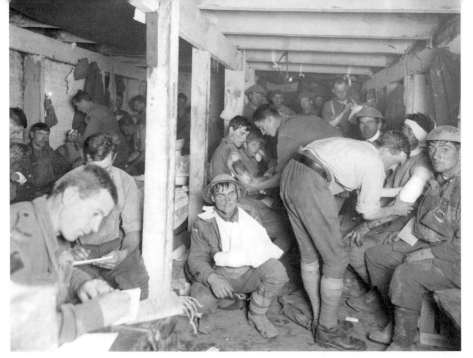

Wounded Australian soldiers being treated in an advanced dressing station in a fortified dugout on the Menin Road near Ypres, Belgium, 20 September 1917. (AWM E00715)

sought escape from the conditions by desertion to the enemy lines, self-inflicted wounds and even suicide.[52] Charles Bean recorded an incident in which a soldier who had run through heavy artillery barrages to deliver messages to a divisional headquarters on 24 July could no longer stand the strain of gunfire; he lay down in the headquarters, put his rifle to his head and shot himself.[53]

British regimental medical officer Charles Wilson described an incident in 1914 when a brooding sergeant, left to rest in billets at Armentières when his unit moved into the trenches, 'blew his head off'. Wilson believed such men 'were unable, not unwilling' and could not face the strain of the trenches. He tortured himself with the question of whether it was right as a medical officer to force them to serve in the trenches, and 'if they were killed were they or I to blame?'[54]

By late 1916, the fighting strength of some Australian battalions fell to fewer than 300 men.[55] Yet still there was worse to come as the Somme winter brought the most severe climate to France in 40 years.[56] Bean considered this period 'the bottom of the curve': over 20,000 Australian soldiers were evacuated with trench feet, frostbite and exhaustion.[57] In the freezing conditions men suffered acutely in the exposed trenches and many prayed for the honourable escape of a 'Blighty' wound or sickness that would force their evacuation. Some deliberately exposed themselves to enemy fire, refusing to take cover from shell explosions. 'I hope I get a decent knock that will send me home again to Blighty,' wrote one soldier in his diary; he had earlier won a Military Medal for bravery in the field.[58]

But the Australian formations recovered, were rebuilt and made notable contributions in the fighting of 1917 and the victorious battles of 1918. The incidence of self-inflicted wounds, as measured by the medical statistics, did not diminish during this period. In fact, reported self-maiming cases were actually more prevalent during the Australian soldiers' most effective phase during the advance to victory in 1918, at more than double the number of the previous two years combined.[59] This is a paradox that awaits further research.

One soldier's experience epitomised the tragedy of men caught on the treadmill of the war in these years. A corporal of the Australian 35th Battalion was arraigned before a District Court Martial in London on 5 February 1919, charged with wilfully maiming himself by shooting himself in the left hand while in the front-line trenches at Villers-Bretonneux on 3 April 1918. The soldier appeared to be both a malingerer and a deserter. He had been declared an 'illegal absentee' after absenting himself without leave in Killarney, Ireland, on 17 August 1918, until he surrendered himself in uniform at AIF Headquarters in London on 25 November 1918.

The president and members of his court martial were all AIF officers. They seemed to take little account of the fact that this soldier had been wounded in action twice on the Western Front, including a gunshot wound to the chest received in the final Australian assault at Passchendaele in October 1917. Both wounds resulted in his evacuation to hospital in England. A doctor who treated him at Killarney Workhouse, to which he had been admitted on 17 May 1918, reportedly suffering from fits and a spinal injury, testified that the soldier 'was suffering from sleeplessness as a result of a shock, presumably shell shock'. The accused man also stated that he 'was suffering from nerves at the end of March' before he went back into the front line at Villers-Bretonneux, although he denied shooting

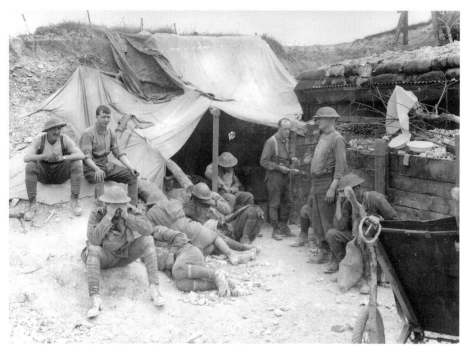

Australian soldiers suffering from the effects of gas, awaiting treatment at a Regimental Aid Post near Villers-Bretonneux, Somme region, France, 27 May 1918. (AWM E04850)

himself, either wilfully or negligently. At the time of his trial, he had served 2 years and 8 months with the AIF (including eight months in France) and, despite two previous minor offences (being found in the sergeants' mess, and absence from parades, for which he was reprimanded), he had not been convicted previously by either a court martial or a civil court.[60]

The court martial found him not guilty of the two charges of self-inflicted wounds but guilty of absence without leave. He was sentenced to 6 months' detention and to be reduced to the ranks. He was admitted to the AIF Detention Barracks at Lewes in Sussex, England, on 21 March 1919 but was discharged just one month later on 25 April 1919 and the remainder of his sentence was remitted.[61]

Almost 80 years later, this soldier's sad story had a poignant aftermath. In July 1998, during commemorative anniversary ceremonies at Fromelles and Hamel in France, the French government announced its intention to confer France's highest honour, the *Légion d'honneur*, on surviving allied veterans who had served on French soil in the First World War. The award was conferred on four Australian veterans

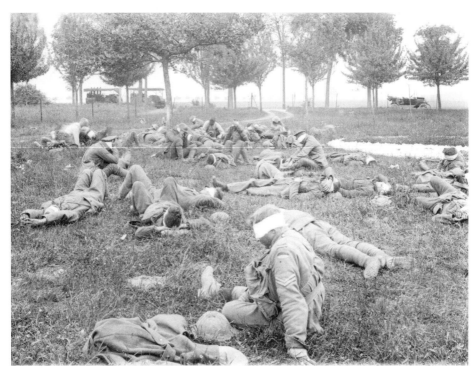

Gassed Australian soldiers awaiting treatment at an overcrowded aid post near Bois de l'Abbé on the Somme, France, 27 May 1918. (AWM E04851)

who visited France at that time and on a further 60 in Australia subsequently. However, three veterans, including this man, were precluded from the award because their service records revealed they had been court-martialled for breaches of military discipline. This particular veteran died two days after Anzac Day in 1999, aged 104 and perhaps never aware that, despite his active service and his wounding in action on the Western Front, he had been refused the belated award.

This soldier was one of the millions of men, volunteers and conscripts, who served in the vast national armies of the Great War. Confronted by the horrors of war in the trenches, they faced the choice between random death and mutilation or the harsh consequences of disobedience. Some who served bravely became reluctant warriors and wounded themselves to escape. As an unknown dimension of the military experience of the First World War, the story of the men who made that desperate choice deserves to be told.

Scarred by war: medical responses
to facially disfigured soldiers
of the Great War

Kerry Neale

In late 2007, Australian Sergeant Michael Lyddiard was deployed with the 3rd Reconstruction Task Force to Afghanistan. While conducting a route clearance task on 2 November, he was seriously wounded when an improvised explosive device he was attempting to render safe detonated. Along with the loss of the lower right arm, he also suffered severe facial wounds and the loss of his right eye. Lyddiard is just one of the many soldiers who have suffered facial disfigurement in recent conflicts such as those in Afghanistan and Iraq. The protection once afforded by trenches during the Great War may now have been replaced by Kevlar body armour, but the face is still left vulnerable. [1]

In June 1918, almost 90 years prior to Lyddiard's wounding, Sir William Arbuthnot Lane, director of the Cambridge Military Hospital at Aldershot, United Kingdom, was quoted in the *New York Times*, saying of facial wound cases:

It's the poor devils without noses and jaws, the unfortunates of the trenches who come back without the faces of men that form the most depressing part of the work … people who look like some of these creatures haven't much of a chance.[2]

But through the dedication and pioneering efforts of British and Dominion surgeons and medical staff, such a chance was to be provided – a chance for these soldiers, and the societies to which they would return, to cope with the brutal damage wrought upon their faces. While Arbuthnot Lane may have considered them to be the 'unfortunates of the trenches', the facially wounded of the Great War could also be considered extremely fortunate with regard to the medical advances being made at this time in the field of maxillofacial reconstructive surgery (that is, reconstruction of the jaw and face).

The Great War changed the lives of thousands of British and Dominion soldiers through disfiguring facial wounds. Unlike other disabilities and wounds – the ones that could be concealed by prosthetics and clothing – facial disfigurement was the most visible and the least concealable type of wound. The loss of a limb from war service came to be seen as a symbol of great patriotism and sacrifice. The disfigurement of a soldier's face, however, does not seem to have been considered in the same way.

The social stigma surrounding facial disfigurement has long been recognised. Writing on facially disfigured veterans from the Napoleonic Wars almost a century earlier, Carl Ferdinand von Graef observed:

We have compassion when we see people on crutches; being crippled does not stop them from being happy and pleasant in society … [But those] who have suffered a deformation of the face, even if it is partially disguised by a mask, create disgust in our imagination.[3]

Perhaps it was because of this stigma or indeed, 'disgust,' that the experiences of disfigured veterans from Britain and the Dominions have been significantly overlooked in social, medical and military histories for the last 90 years. How these veterans dealt with their disfigurement compared with other wounded veterans, and how society responded to them as a unique group of veterans are questions which still remain unanswered.

Facial wounds were extremely common during the Great War – primarily owing to the nature of modern, static warfare, where a soldier's head was particularly vulnerable when exposed above the trench parapet. Even steel helmets, which offered some protection against penetration of the skull, could inflict serious damage themselves when hit, with the resulting metal fragments becoming piercing pieces of shrapnel.

Arthur Graham Butler, the Australian medical historian, claims that of the 312,101 gunshot wounds suffered by Australian soldiers on Gallipoli and the Western Front, and in Egypt and the Middle East, 37,754 (or approximately 12 per cent) were to the head and eyes.[4] Joanna Bourke in her work *Dismembering the Male* (1996) states that British forces suffered more than 60,500 head wounds (approximately 20 per cent of all gunshot wounds).[5] Jay Winter has estimated that approximately 280,000 combatants from Britain, France and Germany were facially wounded, and that as many as one-third of these were permanently disfigured to some degree.[6]

While the Crimean War and American Civil War had given some indication of the horrific nature of facial wounds in modern war, by the time of the Great War, medical technology had not advanced to the same level as the technology of destruction.[7] The increasing use of motor vehicles, however, combined with improving medical treatment being available in the field, meant that many soldiers who would have previously died from such wounds were now surviving and requiring further treatment.

For many facially wounded men, their first hurdle was simply convincing stretcher-bearers that they were worth taking to a Casualty Clearing Station (CCS) or Advanced Dressing Station (ADS). In a memoir written in August–December 1918 (and revised in 1920), British Private Percy Clare describes the moments after he felt a blow to the right side of his face: '[T]here was no pain whatever, and I hardly felt it. But at the same time a stream of blood spouted like a fountain from my mouth and gushed from my nostrils.' A passing soldier tried to use his field dressing kit to staunch the bleeding, but 'in his panic not being able to discover the nature of the wound, only a fountain of blood sprouting from my mouth he stuffed the whole packet in just as it was between my teeth – like a biscuit given to a dog!'[8] Later another soldier tried to bring Clare to the attention of stretcher-bearers. The first stretcher-bearer party to attend Clare thought that, judging by the amount of blood caked on his uniform, he must have a stomach wound. Clare remembered hearing the corporal in charge of the party say that it wouldn't be worth carrying him all that distance as 'that sort always dies soon'.[9]

> A second party my friend brought along also refused me. I was so soaked with blood and looked so sorry a case that they probably were justified that their long tramp with so unpromising a burden would be futile. My persevering friend brought up yet a third party and this time when I roused I found them lifting me on to their stretcher.[10]

Once removed from the battlefield, the second battle for these men would begin – the fight to reconstruct their faces. This second battle began with a slow, painful, and often dangerous journey from a CCS or ADS to a hospital. As with many of the wounded, shock, blood loss and sepsis resulted in death before they even arrived at a hospital. Given the specific nature of their wounds, however, it was essential that the facially wounded travel upright: many would suffocate if they lay down. In the early months of the war, being unaware of this complication, well-meaning nurses and orderlies would help facially wounded soldiers lie back to rest. Often this resulted in the soldier's tongue rolling back in his throat, or blood and mucus blocking his airways. Many went days without food or even water in some cases, owing to the state of their mouths and throats.[11]

Accounts by nursing staff give some indication of what an ordeal being transported was for these soldiers. Many nurses were impressed by their resilience. An anonymous nursing sister wrote in 1914 of her experiences on the medical trains with such cases: 'some of the men, with their eyes, noses or jaws shattered, are so extraordinarily good and uncomplaining'.[12] For others, such as Claire Elise Tisdall, a Voluntary Aid Detachment (VAD) nurse in London, the reaction was shock. A soldier was carried past her at night, and in the dim light she thought that his face was covered with a black cloth, only to realise that the lower half of his face had been blown off and it was a gaping hole. 'That was the only time I nearly fainted [. . .] It was the most frightful sight.'[13] Harold Gillies, who was to treat many of these men at the Queen Mary's Hospital, perhaps best describes what it was like to see these men travelling to the hospitals: 'Men without half their faces; men burned and maimed to the condition of animals. Day after day, the tragic grotesque procession disembarked from the hospital ships and made its way towards us.'[14]

Percy Clare describes his trip on the hospital ship SS *Grantilla Castle*: 'So far except for an external dressing and several inoculations against tetanus, nothing had been, or could be done for my wound.'[15] The first time he was allowed to see his face in a mirror, he 'received rather a shock'.

> My bristly beard was about half an inch long, and dried blood and dirt in it which could only be removed by shaving, looked so disgusting and so altered my appearance that I was quite unhappy [. . .] I was an unlovely object.[16]

Unfortunately, even arrival at a hospital did not guarantee a facial case proper care and treatment. Although he was marked to go to 'special hospital' in London (probably the Cambridge Military Hospital at Aldershot), Clare was instead sent to a hospital at Frensham Hill:

> [It] was a poor sort of place . . . The food was meagre and poor. A mug of tea . . . a doorstep of bread and margarine

constituted our breakfast and was again issued for our tea. There was no provision for such a case as mine: it was 'doorstep' or nothing, and I could not now open my mouth at all. My jaw was swollen and stiff and I had no power to open it. After some difficulty I got porridge and mince included in my diet. The MO told me he wanted me to get up as soon as possible, and get out for walks so that I should get strong enough to travel to a 'special hospital'.[17]

This 'special hospital,' where Clare was eventually to become a patient, was the Queen Mary's Hospital, Sidcup. Word of the remarkable work being undertaken there was soon to provide a sense of comfort to the poor 'unfortunates of the trenches'. One man who was to offer such comfort was Harold Gillies, an ear, nose and throat surgeon from New Zealand.

On August 18, 1917, we moved into Queen's Hospital at Sidcup, and our arrival was simultaneous with a flood of casualties. We literally put down our suitcases and picked up our needle-holders. Is there a better way to open a hospital?[18]

To fully understand the importance of this hospital, it must be put in the context of what had been available previously. In 1916 a specialist maxillofacial unit had been established at the Cambridge Military Hospital, under the command of Gillies. Gillies had joined the British Red Cross at the outbreak of war. In France in 1915 he met Charles August Valadier, who had recently established a special medical unit for treating jaw wounds. Gillies was immediately fascinated by his work. In Paris Gillies later met the French surgeon Hippolyte Morestin, who was also making developments in facial surgery techniques.[19]

After witnessing the work being done by these surgeons and learning of the work of German doctors, Gillies became determined to establish a maxillofacial surgery unit for British imperial forces. In 1916 he arranged for the transfer of all facial wound cases to his small unit at the Cambridge Military Hospital. On his own initiative – and at his own expense – Gillies purchased £10 worth of labels; these directed that the patient onto whose clothing one was pinned should be sent to him at Aldershot. After the battle of the Somme in 1916, the 200 beds available to Gillies at Aldershot fell far short of accommodating the more than 2000 facial wound cases that arrived there. Out of such necessity, the Queen Mary's Hospital was established.[20]

Between its opening in 1917 and its closure in 1925, the surgeons at Queen Mary's Hospital treated over 5000 servicemen from the United Kingdom, the Dominions and the United States, and carried out over 11,000 operations.[21] Gillies hoped that by establishing a specialist institution for the treatment of severe facial wounds, skills and resources could be most effectively used and new techniques could be perfected. The difficulty, as Gillies wrote, was that 'unlike the student . . . who is weaned on small scar excisions and graduates to harelips . . . we were suddenly asked to produce half a face'.[22]

One man given one of Gillies' labels was John Glubb, a British officer who was to become the famous 'Glubb Pasha', commander of the Arab Legion. Glubb was wounded on 21 August 1917 near Arras, France, an event he describes in his memoir, *Into Battle*:

> I think I heard for a second a distant shell whine, then felt a tremendous explosion almost on top of me . . . [T]he floodgates in my neck seemed to burst and the blood poured out in torrents. . . . I could feel something long lying loosely in my left cheek, as though I had a chicken bone in my mouth. It was in reality, half my jaw, which had broken off, teeth and all, and was floating about in my mouth.[23]

Glubb spent no less than three months getting to Sidcup. From the CCS, he was taken to a British Red Cross hospital at Rouen. When he finally sailed for Britain, he should have been taken directly to the Cambridge Military Hospital, as directed by the label he had been issued. But, given the demand on beds there, he was transferred instead to the 3rd London Hospital, Wandsworth. He received no treatment there and his wounds remained septic, not having been re-dressed or cleaned since he left Rouen. Finally, in November 1917, Glubb was transferred to Queen Mary's Hospital, where he received treatment immediately. '[T]hings were very different' there, he observed.[24]

Indeed they were. On 4 August 1917, just prior to the hospital's opening, *The Lancet* published this letter to the editor:

> May we earnestly appeal to the generosity of the public for donations in support of this new hospital for the treatment of many of our most grievously wounded men? This hospital will fulfil a great need. The chief among its objectives being to remove acute cases of facial and jaw injuries from the atmosphere of crowded hospitals into fresh country air and delightful surroundings, and so give these terrible wounds every chance to heal more rapidly [. . .] also to provide cheerful outdoor occupation for the men who frequently have to remain under treatment for 18 months to two years, and who suffer acutely from mental depression.[25]

From the start, Sidcup was to occupy a unique position as a military hospital which had a great deal of support and patronage from the general public, and which provided these men, many of whom underwent more than a dozen operations, not only with medical treatment but also with the psychological support necessary to deal with such trauma. There appears to have been no pressure to return these men to the front to continue fighting; instead, many spent up to two, in some cases even four years undergoing treatment.

Although begun primarily as a British endeavour, Queen Mary's Hospital rapidly took on an imperial feel with staff and surgeons from Australia, New Zealand, Canada, and later, a small unit from America. Gillies commanded the British section; Major C.W. Waldron and Captain Ernest Fulton Risdon at various times commanded the Canadian Section; the New Zealand Section was commanded by Major Henry Percy Pickerill; and Lieutenant Colonel Henry Newland, commanded the Australian Section.[26]

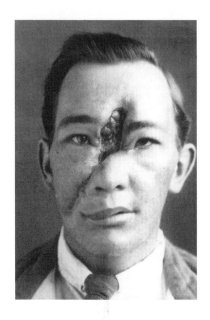

Horrific head and face wounds were a common result of trench warfare in the First World War. Australian Private William Kearsey, photographed on 26 November 1917, was severely wounded by a shell fragment on the Western Front the previous month. He underwent over 20 operations during his 18-month-long treatment at Sidcup hospital in England, before returning to Australia in June 1919. (Image courtesy of the Royal Australasian College of Surgeons.)

The bringing together of such a collection of surgeons from Britain and the Dominions was not a matter of chance, or even of simple convenience. Instead of using specialist surgeons to deal with just one part of the face, the aim was to train and develop well-rounded facial surgeons, who could replace a nose as easily as repair a jaw. Arbuthnot Lane had also realised that the hospital could be improved by competition: 'This competition brought out many men who were excellent at plastic surgery and who also vied with each other in advancing this special form of surgery. The results of their activities were remarkable.'[27] Gillies himself commented on this competitive atmosphere:

> With our artistic efforts constantly on exhibition about the wards, not only the patients judged our results but we, too, if only out of the corners of our eyes, jealously compared our work with that of our colleagues . . . Competition was keen, for the game was on.[28]

Aside from Gillies, the other big player was Henry Pickerill, head of the New Zealand section, who was born in Britain but moved to New Zealand in 1907 to take up the position of director at the newly established Dental School at the University of Otago, Dunedin.

Pickerill was a major in the New Zealand Army Medical Corps and in March 1917 had been appointed to establish a jaw department at the Second New Zealand General Hospital at Walton-on-Thames, near London. Pickerill was reluctant to make the move to Sidcup, but in early 1918 he and his staff, along with 29 of his patients, were transferred to Sidcup. It did not take long for Pickerill to become heavily involved in the work of the hospital; once he saw the state of the men arriving, he quickly became motivated by an intense sense of responsibility. Pickerill commented in the *New Zealand Dental Journal* in July 1918 that he found the work 'exceedingly interesting, making new noses, new lips, ears or eyelids, and bone grafting, all from the patients' own tissues. It is the more fascinating because it is all pioneer work, and one has to think out and devise each case for oneself.'[29]

Indeed, both Pickerill and Gillies were aware of how important it was going to be for the development of facial surgery that each attempted operation or technique be well documented. A number of artists were commissioned to work at Sidcup, and Gillies even took drawing lessons himself, by correspondence, to be better able to record and plan procedures. Professor Henry Tonks, a Slade artist who had worked with Gillies at Aldershot, had described Gillies' unit as 'a chamber of horrors' in a letter to a friend.[30] One can only imagine how he found the scene at Sidcup when he rejoined Gillies there.

Australian artist Lieutenant Daryl Lindsay began working with Gillies and Newland at Sidcup in 1918.[31] While Lindsay was fascinated with the medical innovations being made, he was concerned about his ability to 'translate what looked like a mess of flesh and blood into a diagram a medical student could understand'.[32] To those with no medical training, these diagrams are invaluable in understanding the procedures undergone by these patients. The paintings serve as a colour record of the men's wounds, and reveal the extent of the damage and disfiguration in a realistic manner that is often more confronting than the black-and-white photographs.

One of the groundbreaking techniques developed by Gillies was the pedicle tube. In this procedure the patient's own flesh was cut then curled to form a tube that would allow for the skin to be

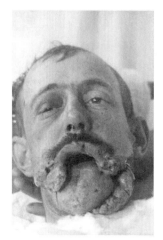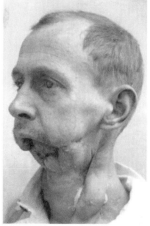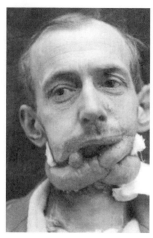

Stages in the reconstruction of the severely damaged lower jaw of Australian Private Eric Winter, admitted to Sidcup hospital in October 1917. Surgeons secured his tongue with skin grafts and grafted pedicle tubes from his upper chest to the jaw. Photographs dated (from left) 24 October 1917, 18 July 1918, 2 February 1919. (Images courtesy of the Royal Australasian College of Surgeons.)

grafted on while maintaining a continuous flow of blood to the area. Gillies himself referred to the discovery of the technique as 'a major break-through'.[33] The treatment of Australian private, Eric Winter, demonstrated an extensive use of this technique for the repair of the lower jaw. Winter was admitted to Sidcup on 22 October 1917, with only a small piece of his lower lip remaining on the right-hand side and a gaping wound on his right cheek.[34] In January of the following year, grafts of skin from under Winter's jaw were brought to his upper lip to draw in his chin and secure his tongue in its cavity. In July 1918, a pedicle tube was grafted on: it ran from the upper chest to the side of the lower jaw. By February 1919, the pedicle tubes were transferred from his upper chest to the area of the lower jaw. No further details are available from Winter's file.[35]

Administering anaesthetic to patients with faces as badly damaged as Winter's presented a distinct problem. The usual method of administering anaesthetic during this period involved placing chloroform cloths over the mouth and nose of the patient or blowing ether vapour into a funnel covering his face. This often meant that the surgeons themselves were affected by the vapour exhaled by the unconscious patient; furthermore, the need for the funnel made it almost impossible to use this method in facial surgery. It was only through the work of the Irish anaesthetist Ivan Magill that such difficulties were overcome. Magill developed a method whereby a tube was inserted through the nose or mouth directly into the patient's lungs, thus allowing the surgeon access to the areas to be worked on.[36]

In some cases surgery could only do so much, and other means of repair, or rather concealment, had to be used. Rifleman Moss had been blinded when he lost both eyes. He was fitted with a prosthetic mask to conceal, at least partially, his disfigurement. The mask was kept in place by a pair of glasses, to which it was attached. Moss provides one example of a case where it appears it was considered somehow more acceptable to be blind than disfigured. As Gillies put it: 'Fitted with an external prosthesis, at least [Moss] was presentable enough to become a blind man.'[37] Quite often, facial wounds could also result in partial or total loss of sight, and Gillies observed that at Sidcup 'only the blind kept their spirits up through thick and thin'.[38]

Mirrors were prohibited in the wards at Sidcup. This way sighted patients could be spared the shock of seeing themselves as they underwent their numerous operations. It also meant that staff could better control the process whereby patients were shown their changed appearance. However, many of the men found ways around this. A quick survey of the men around them would have given most patients an idea of the state of their own faces, and catching a glimpse of their reflection in a window could also be traumatic. Catherine Black, a nursing sister who had worked with Gillies at Aldershot, described one corporal's reaction to seeing himself:

To my dismay I found a corporal in possession of [a mirror] that evening. None of us had even known he had a shaving glass in his locker. I pretended not to see it when he called me over and asked me to pull the screens round his bed. Every nurse learns that there are moments when it is better to leave a patient alone, because sympathy would only make matters worse. I think he must have fought out his battle in the night, for early next morning he asked for pen and paper and wrote a letter to Molly [his sweetheart]. 'You're well

enough to see her now,' I said. 'Why not let her come down?'
'She will never come now,' he said quietly, and there was the
finality of despair in his voice.[39]

One can only imagine how distressing the situation must have been,
both for staff and patients. The nature of the men's wounds meant
that, for most, speech was very limited, if not impossible, and that
eating was also a difficult and painful experience. Often soup and
milk would have to be poured down a tube inserted into the patient's
throat. His mouth then had to be sluiced with water to keep it clean
and reduce the chance of infection.[40]

The inability to communicate would have been a source of great
frustration for many of these patients, as would the feeling of being
reduced to an almost child-like dependency on the nursing staff. A
diagnosis of depression was never recorded in any of the patients'
medical files. Nevertheless, Gillies noticed how, in cases at both
Sidcup and Aldershot, 'if we made a poor repair for a wretched
fellow the man's character was inclined to change for the worse. He
would become morose, break rules and give trouble generally.'[41] But
when they 'made a good repair, the patient usually became a happy
convalescent and soon regained his old character and habits.'[42]

Some patients even managed to find humour in being consulted
on the repair of their features. Gillies often made his own suggestions
as to how a patient's features could be best restored; the joke being
that he could even improve on their pre-war appearance. Horace
Sewell recalls the day that he was consulted on the repair to his nose:

I still see the friendly smile that gave us so much confidence
in him [Gillies]. His greeting one morning was, 'Well,
Paddy, your big day is here. What sort of nose do you think
we ought to give you?' He made various sketches of me . . .
with different shaped noses. 'I'm not fussy, sir.' I said, and he
decided I should have a Roman nose, as my face was rather
round.[43]

Some, however, decided to make do with the features their misfortune had left them with. John Glubb, for example, was shown an album of 'photographs of handsome young men and asked to choose the chin I would like to have!' On learning how long it would take to build this new chin, he decided to 'retain my old face, or whatever was left of it'.[44]

While Arbuthnot Lane may have considered these men to be the 'unfortunates of the trenches,' Gillies described his 'wounded boys' as 'a brave lot'.[45] The dedication of the surgeons, and the importance they placed on aesthetics as well as function, undoubtedly provided these men with their best chance of reconstructing not only their faces, but also their lives. Although it was certainly not an easy process, Gillies believed that 'once we started their repair their morale usually led the pace, as evidenced by many a moustache perking up with a bit of spit and twist'.[46] What is certain is that these 'unfortunates of the trenches' proved to be most fortunate in receiving some of the best treatment for facial wounds available at the time.

'The home is always here for him': disabled soldiers and family caregiving in Australia after the First World War

Marina Larsson

In 1927 Mrs Clara Stephens wrote to the repatriation authorities requesting an increased war pension for her son. Herbert Stephen had returned from the First World War in 1919 suffering from shell shock and became a resident of the Mont Park Repatriation Mental Hospital north of Melbourne. In 1926 his condition improved and he was released into the care of his parents. The Stephens' new life with their 40-year-old son was difficult because he was 'not normal'.[1] He slept erratically and walked about the house at all hours of the day and night. The lives of Clara and her husband, John, were dominated by their son's needs. They fed and clothed him, and helped him manage his mental struggles from day to day. The burdens of home care upon the Stephens were significant and unrelenting, yet they loyally continued to support him, insisting that 'the home is always here for him'. In her letter, Clara informed the Department that she and her husband were struggling to manage Herbert's condition, reflecting 'it has been a long war to us'.[2]

The Stephens family was one of thousands of Australian families who cared for a physically or mentally disabled soldier after the First World War. During the postwar period, the number of families left to support a 'disabled digger' was significantly greater than those who mourned the 'fallen'. Of the 324,000 soldiers who served overseas, more than 60,000 were killed, but a further 90,000 were disabled.[3] To put this in perspective, out of every ten soldiers who served, two were killed and a further three were disabled. While some severely disabled men required permanent institutionalisation, the majority were cared for in their homes by their kin.

This chapter examines the caregiving work of families, like the Stephens, who looked after disabled Australian soldiers after the Great War. It argues that families played a vital role in the repatriation of damaged ex-servicemen, and that their unpaid labour constituted an important tier of welfare that underpinned the formal repatriation system. Yet both during and after the war, families received little official or public acknowledgement of their efforts. As one observer noted in 1918, family caregiving was 'the part we do not see'.[4] Caregiving occurred within the domestic sphere and it was rarely documented or written about by Repatriation Department officials or public commentators. This lack of documentation is frustrating. However, it is also productive, for it prompts us to ask why families received such little recognition for their domestic labours, given the importance and prevalence of their work in the 1920s and 1930s.

Historians have been slow to examine the role of families in the care, treatment and convalescence of disabled soldiers after the First World War. Family caregiving still remains 'the part we do not see'. This is understandable. Historians tend to write about what we find in the archives. As Jay Winter has noted in the British context, although we know that it was often family members who shouldered the burden of care, 'virtually all' of this work went unrecorded.[5] What we do find in the archives is evidence about the medical treatment, rehabilitation, pensioning and the vocational training of disabled soldiers. Current histories of war disability faithfully reflect these sources, with many scholars drawing out the cultural and gendered dimensions of disablement, for individual men and groups such as the limbless, the blind and the shell-shocked.

Yet families' experiences of war disability are strikingly absent from the historical literature. This is curious, given that since the 1980s, historians of mental illness such as Roy Porter, Mark Finnane and David Wright have opened the door to writing new kinds of histories, which explore the interconnected worlds of physicians, patients and their families in the context of state and private medical care.[6] In this literature, which draws mostly on nineteenth-century archives, family members are the 'new historical actors', whose role in sickness care – as Roy Porter reminds us – should not be underestimated.[7] By contrast, within the world of military medical history, 'care' is still primarily viewed as a consequence of the relationship between the soldier and the state, rather than between the soldier and his family.[8]

During the war, the first disabled soldiers returned to Australia in mid-1915. They and the thousands who followed them had sustained a diverse range of disabilities. Modern warfare literally 'shattered' the male body. Although the limbless soldier became an iconic wartime image, fewer than 3500 soldiers returned without a limb.[9] In reality, most injuries took the form of invisible internal damage to organs, bones, muscles and other bodily systems. As the war progressed, increasing numbers of men were invalided home with 'shell shock'. While some severely impaired men became long-term patients in repatriation facilities, most returned home after medical treatment had ceased.

Although the hospital looms large in how we imagine the care of disabled soldiers to have been conducted, home was the cornerstone of this care for most men. Indeed, most ex-servicemen, if given the choice, stated the Limbless and Maimed Soldiers' Association in 1920, preferred 'to remain with their wife and family' rather than reside at the 'Repat'.[10] These men joined a much larger population of civilian disabled being cared for in their family homes. Despite the rise of hospital and institutional care in the nineteenth and early twentieth centuries, the home was still the most significant site of care for the disabled and chronically ill in the Edwardian era, for soldier and civilian alike.[11]

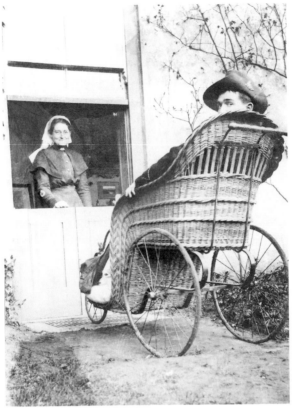

Matron Ethel Gray of the Australian Army Nursing Service watching over an Australian soldier patient in a cane wheelchair at No. 1 Australian Auxiliary Hospital, Harefield, England, in 1916. (AWM P02402.013)

In order to talk about family caregiving, we first need to build up a picture of soldiers' family circumstances. The First AIF was overwhelmingly made up of young men: 52 per cent of them were aged between 18 and 24, and 80 per cent were unmarried.[12] This means that, in the first instance, the primary caregivers of disabled soldiers were their parents. Indeed, some disabled men never married because of their disabilities and remained in the care of their parents well into the 1930s. Many disabled men, however, did successfully marry and form their own families. During and after the war, single women were encouraged by patriotic publications to marry the war disabled, and embrace their feminine role as nurturers and carers. In 1918 the *Everylady's Journal* advised one young woman to think of her disabled fiancé 'wounded, body, soul, and spirit – as you would think of a little child … [and] with your most tender care win [him] back to happier ways, to brighter thoughts, this returned broken man'.[13] After marrying a disabled soldier, some wives faced a life of caregiving: they quite literally looked after their husbands 'in sickness and in health'.

Within the home, the caregiving activities of family members were diverse, and varied according to the nature and extent of their soldier's impairments and how his health fluctuated over time. Notably the labours of kin were gendered. Wives, mothers and sisters most commonly became the providers of nursing care, which reflected women's responsibility in the early twentieth century for the management and emotional sustenance of the household.[14] Women carers ensured that medicines were correctly administered, and they prepared special remedies and health-giving foods.[15] In some instances, the nursing care they provided was not only intimate but confronting. In mid-1917 Mrs Louisa Hogan commenced a regimen of hand-feeding her son with liquid meals. Frederick Hogan had returned home with his 'lower jaw shot away' and was unable to use his right arm.[16]

While direct-care responsibilities typically fell to women, a range of family members provided other forms of support. Fathers offered practical assistance, such as providing transport to hospital appointments, dealing with the repatriation bureaucracy or taking mobility-impaired men on excursions. Other relatives were called upon to provide company for bedridden men who, as one departmental official observed, had 'nothing to do' and relied heavily upon their family members for entertainment.[17]

Within the home, shell-shocked soldiers made up one of the most challenging groups for which families cared. As the *RSA Magazine* observed in 1919, the wives and mothers of such men required 'an unusual degree of unselfish devotion'.[18] The repatriation medical records of Albert Brown reveal that by the late 1920s, his wife was struggling in her role as his primary carer. Albert had returned to Melbourne from Gallipoli with physical wounds, and upon arriving home his mental outlook also began to decline. He became subject to 'moody turns' and 'would sometimes sit for hours without speaking'.[19] Mrs Brown tried to be supportive of her husband, but when he developed paranoid thoughts, she asked Albert's sister, May, to move into the household. By that stage Albert required around-the-clock monitoring, which could only be achieved with two live-in carers.[20] The endeavours of Mrs Brown and May suggest that there may have been a shortage of beds in a repatriation mental institution, which had become overcrowded by the late 1920s. It may also indicate they were trying to avoid Albert's institutionalisation, which many families experienced as shameful owing to the stigma of mental illness and having to enter an 'asylum'. They did so by ensuring that he remained in his own home for as long as possible.

Like Mrs Brown, the carers of disabled soldiers often called upon relatives to ease their burden of care. Sisters, aunts and resident grandmothers all undertook various domestic responsibilities to release primary caregivers. Families were networks of survival for disabled soldiers, and the willingness of a greater number of family members to help was an advantage. Conversely, disabled soldiers with smaller families or strained relationships had fewer opportunities to share the load. As well as providing home-based care, nuclear and extended families also offered their loved ones economic support. Some men did not receive sufficient pension income to support their families, and struggled to get a suitable job in the mainstream workforce. In some instances, wives supported their husbands to establish cottage industries at home, such as poultry farming. Other families found a role for men within existing family businesses. During the 1920s Harold Kenworthy, a tubercular soldier, was employed by his uncle on the understanding that he could take plenty of time off for ill health.[21]

While the family was a site of caregiving for many disabled soldiers, it is important to remember that kin support was not available to all returned men. A number of families were unwilling to take on the demands of caregiving, or found that their capacity to provide support changed as the years passed. During the 1920s, Robert Mundey's anti-social behaviour was so extreme that his family was no longer able to care for him at home.[22] Having enlisted at the age of just 16, Robert was discharged suffering from the effects of gunshot wounds, gassing and shell shock. After his discharge, he took to drinking and began to exhibit violent and erratic behaviour. By 1926 he was camping alone in a hut, unable to secure appropriate accommodation or support from his family.[23] In some instances, the absence of family carers meant that the responsibility of care fell to friends. In 1919, after the death of his mother, Charles Berg, a paralysed soldier from Sydney, was taken in by close friends of the family, Mr and Mrs Semple, who subsequently showed him 17 years of 'unremitting kindness'.[24]

The sacrifices made by family members to support disabled ex-servicemen often came at a personal cost. War 'disabled' the lives of kin as well as soldiers. One blinded ex-serviceman noted that women's 'own health must suffer' as a result of supporting a dependent disabled husband.[25] Indeed, under the strain, some women simply did not cope. In May 1918 the distraught mother of a severely disabled Rutherglen soldier committed suicide, unable to deal with her son's extensive disability.[26] After many years of caregiving, a number of families simply abandoned their sons and husbands to institutions. In 1930 Mrs Dorothy Clements asked the authorities whether she could 'go into the country with her children' because she felt that she could no longer 'do anything' for her husband, a shell-shocked veteran in a Melbourne mental hospital.[27]

The 1930s was a particularly difficult decade for these families. As the Great Depression hit, ageing disabled ex-servicemen found themselves unable to compete in a shrinking labour market. Moreover, the Scullin government cut families' war disability allowances by 22.5 per cent as part of its Financial Emergency Act. Sometimes unemployment and financial troubles precipitated a nervous breakdown, particularly among shell-shocked men whose psychological state was already fragile. Parents and wives, many of whom had provided support to their soldier for years, were themselves growing older and frailer. Mrs Clara Stephens's letter to the Repatriation Department in 1927 indicates the plight of ageing parents who were still looking after their middle-aged sons: '(my husband) is 73 years and I am 65 years', she wearily declared, as she described her son's erratic behaviour.[28]

Despite the burdens carried by soldiers' kin, family-based

caregiving received little official recognition by the Repatriation Department. One reason for this was that the Australian repatriation system was based on a formal administrative relationship between the government and the individual soldier, rather than his family unit.[29] Under the Australian Soldiers' Repatriation Act, officials were not obliged to document, comment upon or monitor the welfare of those who were officially classified as veterans' 'dependants'. The caregiving work of family members, then, was administratively invisible within a model which conceptualised war disability as a problem for individual servicemen, rather than as a family issue.

This sentiment reflected a broader idea within contemporary rehabilitation literature that the proper role of kin was to 'stand behind' the disabled soldier and help him recover his independence.[30] In 1922 one British rehabilitation manual even suggested that 'sympathising relatives and friends' actually lessened men's chances of success in civilian life.[31] Within departmental literature, and also in public domain sources, war disability was most commonly written about in a narrative of individual men's personal struggle and triumph. In this literature, disabled soldiers fought their 'second battle' alone, without needing help from kin.

This reluctance to publicly discuss disabled soldiers' reliance on family caregivers reflected a social stigma around male dependence. During the early twentieth century, male dependence was antithetical to the dominant codes of masculinity. It undercut the ideal of the manly breadwinner, and the version of manhood espoused by the ANZAC legend, which revolved around the lone, resilient and self-reliant digger. The reluctance to discuss family members' burdens can also be attributed to an unwillingness to publicly undercut the battlefield sacrifices of soldiers by highlighting the domestic sacrifices of their kin. Yet, the dominant public image of the disabled soldier – a 'familyless' individual on the road to manly independence – was an ideal at odds with the lives of most ex-servicemen.

Although the Australian Soldiers' Repatriation Act of 1917 ushered in a new and revolutionary era in the history of the Australian welfare state, the repatriation system did not replace the family as a key provider of care and support for ex-servicemen. During and after the First World War, families remained a primary locus of emotional, social and economic support. The dependence of disabled soldiers on their kin was not the exception: it was commonplace. Under the Act, family members were officially designated as 'dependants' of ex-servicemen. Paradoxically, however, veterans were often dependent on their kin.

The skilled unpaid caregiving labour of family members formed a publicly invisible second repatriation system, without which the nation would never have 'recovered' from war. The type of support offered by kin was unique to each family and of a highly personal and responsive nature that arguably could never have been replicated by state agencies. The stories of these families remind us that repatriation was not only a state-managed process which facilitated the integration of soldiers back into civilian life, but a personal journey which took place within the private haven of the home and was negotiated within the context of familial relationships.

To conclude, I want to suggest that our medical histories of the First World War, or any war for that matter, are not complete without recognising the extent and significance of family caregiving. Families' experiences of care have been shared and passed down *within* veterans' own family networks; however, they continue to occupy a peripheral place in the mainstream histories of war. That is because, with some exceptions, our histories tend to be soldier- and physician-centred. I am by no means saying that classically framed medical and military histories should not be written. I would suggest, however, that there needs to be a greater awareness of the role of families in the care, treatment and convalescence of returned soldiers, as well as families' partnerships with physicians and other care providers.

Without recognising families' contribution to soldiers' repatriation, our history is not complete. The family was a key site of repatriation for disabled soldiers. But writing this history is easier said than done. Researching family caregiving is challenging. Written archival sources are few and far between. During and after the

First World War, physicians and hospitals generated a wealth of records which today are a goldmine for medical historians. By contrast, families had little reason to record their caregiving activities. Official repatriation medical records do not comprehensively document family life, and public commentators were largely silent on the subject. Indeed, the bureaucratic structures of the 'Repat', which were organised around the individual soldier, obscure our present-day view of the private structures of support that ex-servicemen found within their own homes.

The history of caregiving exists in the margins of case files and within families' own collective memories. To uncover their experiences, we need to listen to the 'silences' in the archives, engage with the oral histories of descendants, and read their family photos as historical documents about war disability. We need to explore the human relationships that sustained veterans: not simply trace the pensions paper trail. To gain a glimpse into the domestic realm, we must read – 'against the grain', as it were – soldiers' medical files, official literature and public commentary for traces of their 'dependants' as whole people. In practical terms, this can mean trawling through 20 or 30 case files before finding one letter from a soldier's wife or mother, and then going to other local and family archives to build up a picture of family life with reference to non-military sources.

Writing a family-centred history of the 'wounds of war' means writing about relationships and shared experiences, and recognising the porous boundaries between hospital and home. It means putting the family at the centre of research, even when written archives, at first glance, appear to tell us only about soldiers and doctors.

Rabbit war wounds

Paul Weindling

In January 1942 SS *Obergruppenführer* Reinhard Heydrich, the head of the Reich Security Office, convened the Wannsee Conference to formalise plans for the 'Final Solution of the Jewish Problem'. A few months later, this archetype of the SS clan warrior was the target of a daring assassination mission, aimed to show that Nazi leaders could have no immunity from retribution. On 27 May 1942 two parachutists from the Czech Brigade in Britain ambushed and wounded Heydrich – who was acting Protector of Bohemia and Moravia – on the outskirts of Prague in 'Operation Anthropoid'.[1] Heydrich, who had reached for his gun and chased his assailants, was expected to recover. Sudeten German surgeons from the German University of Prague rapidly operated with apparent success.[2] The bullet hit the rear axle and went up vertically through Heydrich's back, carrying cloth, wire and wool of the car seat. His wounds became infected by gangrene. The bullet prompted Nazi doctors to argue over how best to treat infected wounds. *Reichsführer-SS* Heinrich Himmler (head of the SS) ordered the surgeon Karl Gebhardt, a school friend and his escort surgeon, to Prague to save Heydrich's life.[3] Gebhardt found that the site of the wound and its contamination prevented his operating to remove the damaged spleen. Heydrich died on 4 June.

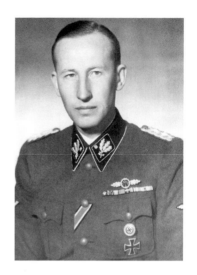

SS Obergruppenführer Reinhard Heydrich, who was head of the Third Reich Security Office and architect of the 'Final Solution of the Jewish Problem'. He died from injuries suffered during an assassination attempt on his life in May 1942. (Image courtesy of bpk, Bildagentur für Kunst, Kultur und Geschicte, 10007641 bpk.)

The Nazi leadership's consternation turned to ruthless revenge with the destruction of the village of Lidice: its men were shot, women were sent to concentration camps, and children were taken for forced adoption. But there was a calculating, medical side to SS brutality, about which the accounts of the Heydrich assassination are generally silent.

Hitler's medical entourage erupted in vicious recrimination. The Führer's doctor, Theo Morrell, criticised Gebhardt for not using what he claimed was his more powerful patent form of sulphonamide, Ultraseptyl. The sulphonamides at first contained the infection, but then rapidly lost their effectiveness.[4] Himmler used the Heydrich incident to gain a hold on military surgery through the SS military branch, the *Waffen-SS*. He authorised Gebhardt and a team of *Waffen-SS* military surgeons to embark on experiments on the legs of concentration-camp prisoners. The surgeons were ambitious to produce a German answer to the British discovery of penicillin, announced in *The Lancet* in August 1940. The first tests on a handful of severe and often fatal infections were published early in 1941.[5] It was a chance for the arrogant Gebhardt to prove that operative skill had greater value than chemotherapy, while exonerating himself from the charge that he was incompetent in letting Heydrich die.

The Nazi takeover drew Gebhardt to the Northern plains of Berlin-Brandenburg. Reich Physicians' *Führer* Gerhard Wagner had

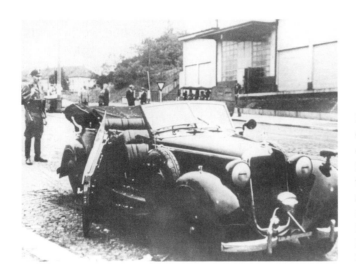

Heydrich's Mercedes car showing the extensive damage it sustained during the assassination attempt on his life. (Image courtesy of bpk, Bildagentur für Kunst, Kultur und Geschicte, 30014457 bpk.)

appointed him on 1 November 1933 director of the rambling Red Cross sanatorium of Hohenlychen. He modernised it as a centre of orthopaedic medicine, emulating the American model of Warm Springs, and founded a medical institute at the Academy of Gymnastics in Berlin. In 1935 Gebhardt transferred to the University of Berlin to develop sports medicine and orthopedics, as professor from 1937.[6] His prestige rose when he took charge of the medical care for Olympic athletes at the Berlin Games of 1936. Sports were an opportunity for orthopedic surgeons to display their mastery of muscular traction.

Himmler and the SS Criminal Police chief Arthur Nebe ordered that wound experiments be carried out in the concentration camp of Ravensbrück.[7] Medical researchers discussed whether it would not be better to monitor therapeutic trials on already infected patients, but Himmler wanted to replicate laboratory conditions in concentration camps.[8] The standard method involved comparing results with the experiences of a control group. There was nothing like a randomised statistical trial.

In the faltering Russian campaign, military surgeons saw the experiments as harnessing German military medical research to combat infections threatening front-line troops. These included hepatitis (which German researchers claimed to be an infectious rather than chronic disease), the insect-borne diseases of typhus and malaria (all widespread in North Africa and on the Eastern front), and wound infections.

Gebhardt organised an SS medical station at Hohenlychen. The *Waffen-SS* took Hohenlychen over in 1941 as part of its expanding realm of medical institutions. Gebhardt inspected *Waffen-SS* field hospitals in Russia,[9] and attained high rank as SS-Gruppenführer and Generalleutnant in the *Waffen-SS*. Hohenlychen was just 12 kilometres from Ravensbrück, and readily accessible from Berlin. The concentration camp was sited in what had been an Olympic village for the 1936 Berlin Olympic Games. Gebhardt was ambitious to develop Hohenlychen into a major centre of experimental medicine with an institute of cancer research. The Allied bombing of Berlin meant that Gebhardt gained a division of the pathology department from that city's Virchow Hospital.[10]

Relative seclusion from Allied bombs meant Hohenlychen became a haunt of Nazi leaders, and conspiracy. Gebhardt treated Hitler's architect and armaments minister Speer, the French Minister of Production Jean Bichelonne, the Nazi agriculturalist Walter Darré, and other prominent politicians. Bichelonne died after his operation and Speer considered that Gebhardt attempted to kill him while under treatment in January to March 1944.[11] Gebhardt sheltered Himmler's mistress, Häschen Potthast (the 'little hare'), who gave birth to their second child at the sanatorium.[12]

Gebhardt ordered Fritz Fischer (who transferred from the Virchow Hospital) to carry out the wounding experiments, and another assistant, Ludwig Stumpfegger, was involved in the bone transplantation experiments.[13] Stumpfegger was appointed in Gebhardt's place to attend Himmler and then in Karl Brandt's place as Hitler's surgeon-in-attendance in October 1944. He remained in the *Führerbunker* until Hitler committed suicide.[14]

In 1942, 15 male prisoners – possibly Russians – were transferred from Sachsenhausen concentration camp on the northern outskirts of Berlin to Ravensbrück for use as experimental subjects.[15] Women prisoners were then favoured as subjects, because of the view that women would be more docile. Seventy-four women fell victim to the experiments and several did not survive. The women were mainly Polish, but there were a few Ukrainians and a Jehovah's Witness.[16]

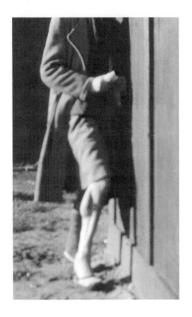

This clandestine photograph of the disfigured leg of Maria Kusmierczuk, a Polish political prisoner in the Ravensbrück concentration camp, was smuggled out by a French prisoner and later published by the Polish underground press. Kusmierczuk was one of many women of the Polish resistance subjected to barbaric medical experiments, including deliberately infected wounds. Terming themselves 'Rabbits' in protest at their treatment, 55 survived despite severe and disabling injuries. (Image courtesy of US Holocaust Memorial Museum, Photograph 69339.)

From 1 August 1942 Gebhardt's underlings selected Polish nationalist resistance fighters as experimental targets. The compliant camp doctor, Herta Oberheuser, declared that the Germans had the right to experiment on these subjects because they were members of the resistance. This was in line with the firmly held German belief, often stated, that their experimental subjects were under a death sentence – this assumed that all camp inmates were guilty by virtue of their imprisonment.

At first, Gebhardt's team surgically wounded the prisoners' legs, but *Reichsarzt* SS Ernst Robert Grawitz ordered that victims' legs be gashed with splinters and glass shards, and infected with tetanus to replicate battlefield conditions.[17] When the Hohenlychen surgeons did not go to this extreme, Himmler was angered that no deaths resulted – the greater the brutality, the more the surgical perpetrators would be bound into the SS. Oberheuser selected camp prisoners with perfectly healthy legs, which had no signs of infection. The Hohenlychen doctors gashed the legs and infected the wounds with wood and glass shards; they broke bones, transplanted them, placed the injured limbs in traction, and destroyed muscles and nerve fibres. Bacteria that could cause gangrene were put into the wounds of one group, and in another cultures causing blood poisoning. In the event, 13 of the 74 experimental subjects died from gangrene and tetanus or from loss of blood, and six were executed. Wladyslawa Karolewska protested against a third operation on her: she objected that 'it was not allowed to perform operations on political prisoners without their consent'. Assisted by solidarity among the victims and their fellow prisoners, 55 survived despite severe and crippling wounds.[18]

The victims turned their sufferings into resistance, and styled themselves 'Rabbits'. In March 1943 they protested in writing to the camp commandant, Fritz Suhren, then refused to attend the Revier (the camp hospital) for further 'experiments'.[19] The Rabbits confronted the camp commandant and demanded that he inform them whether the operations were part of their sentence. In February 1943 they submitted a statement that 'international law does not even permit experimental operations on criminals/ political prisoners'. This was an audacious stance, separating their status as internees from their ordeals as experimental victims. The International Committee of the Red Cross did nothing to halt the medical abuses, and the camp authorities conceded that the experiments went beyond an appropriate punitive regime.[20] It was an epic protest, which the judges at the Nuremberg Medical Trial cited when delivering judgment on Gebhardt, Fischer and Oberheuser.[21]

The Ravensbrück commandant, Suhren, disapproved of the experiments, principally because the prisoners' opposition provoked poor discipline. Suhren declined to hand over further prisoners for experiments. On 15 August 1943 ten prisoners refused to present themselves for more operations. Ten days later Suhren was ordered to report to Richard Glücks (the Inspector of the Concentration Camps) who asked him why he was refusing to supply patients. Glücks accompanied Suhren to Gebhardt in Hohenlychen, where Suhren was humiliatingly forced to apologise. Himmler ordered Suhren to supply three more human guinea pigs. This was the final group of experiments carried out in the camp, and as Suhren foretold, the girls revolted and were operated on by force in the camp prison.[22]

The Rabbits planned to alert the Allies and the Vatican about their plight. One prisoner, Nina Iwanska, had the idea of sending

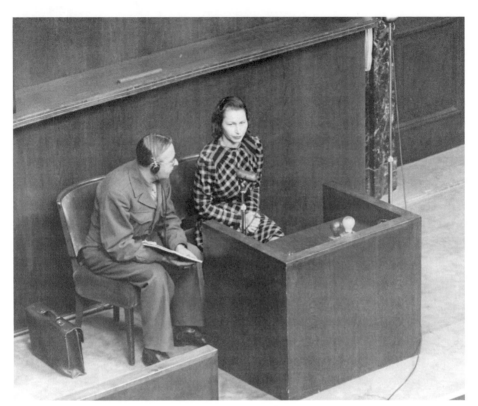

Wladislava Karolewska, one of four Polish women who appeared as prosecution witnesses in 1947 during the Medical Case trial of the Nuremberg Proceedings. Twenty-three German physicians, scientists and officials were charged with war crimes and crimes against humanity for conducting medical experiments on civilian prisoners. (Image courtesy of US Holocaust Memorial Museum, Photograph 43019.)

letters to their families with code words and secret writing in urine. She joined with Krystyna Iwanska, Wanda Wojtasik (a psychiatrist from Cracow), and Krystyna Czyz (a geography teacher from Lublin) in sending messages to their families with details of the 74 Rabbits. [23] They asked that news of these experiments be sent to the BBC in London, the Red Cross in Geneva, a Swiss Catholic mission in Fribourg, and Polish exiles in Lisbon. Labour detachments came into the camp from outside, and communicated details of the atrocities.[24] A French prisoner, Germaine Tillion (later a distinguished anthropologist), secretly carried a roll of undeveloped photographic film with pictures of the injured legs from 21 January 1944 until she left the camp.[25]

The Polish underground press published details of the

experiments, and the Lublin command of a resistance group sent the information to London. The Reich Security Office informed Gebhardt that intelligence about the experiments had reached Great Britain and Switzerland, and a delegate of the actively pro-German Swiss Red Cross told him late in 1944 that the Polish government in exile had condemned him to death.[26] In December 1943 a released prisoner who had US citizenship left the camp with a list of the names of the victims and the dates of the operations.[27] Investigating the events early in 1946, Keith Mant, a British army forensic pathologist, proved that the experiments were not instigated by the camp medical staff but arose from Gebhardt's initiative.[28]

The sulphonamide experiments were part of a broader pattern of human experimentation by the Germans. One can draw a few more general comparative observations:

1. The experiments showed a higher proportion of those who survived to those who were killed.

2. The experiments were mainly on Poles – the largest victim group – although this group divides into Jews and non-Jews.

3. The main target group among women was made up of young adults – exactly as in this experiment. However, men outnumbered women.

4. From a structural perspective the experiments were part of a phase of militarily related experiments. Once the Germans realised that the war was lost the experiments intensified, and the victims became ever younger. There was also a shift to the racially expendable – Jews, and Sinti and Roma (or colloquially gypsies).

5. Prisoner researchers at Auschwitz and Buchenwald duped their German scientific masters, and relished the opportunity for sabotage and delivering bogus results and useless batches of vaccine.[29]

6. These experiments were known to the International

Committee of the Red Cross, which lamentably failed
to assist and intervene on behalf of the victims. More
robust safeguards for civilians under enemy occupation,
and for patients generally, were necessary.

Gebhardt was tried at Nuremberg from December 1946 to August
1947; then convicted and executed. But there was no compensation
or treatment for the victims. The Rabbits became a *cause célèbre* in a
drawn-out battle for compensation that has continued unresolved;
today eleven still survive.

Medical responses to the liberation of Nazi camps, April–May 1945

Debbie Lackerstein

In the final weeks of the Second World War in Europe – in April and May 1945 – American and British units moving rapidly through Germany began to uncover camps that contained thousands of emaciated, diseased and dying people. The inmates were incarcerated in conditions of indescribable filth and overcrowding and with them were thousands of unburied and decomposing corpses. The living and the dead gave evidence of the cruellest neglect and of the most barbaric crimes. The soldiers who first entered the camps and the media units that very soon accompanied them were keen to bear witness to the horror. Many immediately found in the camps the reason and justification for fighting this war at such an immense cost. Yet those who witnessed the liberation, even those who were sent to report it, felt unable to convey the nature of the human tragedy that confronted them. Richard Dimbleby, the BBC war correspondent reporting from Belsen, felt that he could not adequately explain what he saw and told his audience that he would simply give the facts, 'unadorned'.

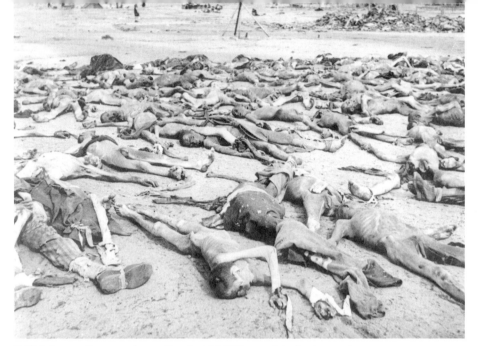

British forces discovered an estimated 10,000 emaciated prisoners'
corpses when they liberated the concentration camp of Belsen in
Germany on 15 April 1945. This scene was recorded by Australian official
war photographer Lieutenant Alan Moore. (AWM P03007.013)

American reporter, Ed Murrow, said in his radio broadcast from
Buchenwald that the best he could do was merely to describe part
what he had seen and heard: 'For most of it,' he said 'I have no words.'[1]

These initial responses to the liberation of the camps attest to the
tremendous shock of discovery. But they also show that the Western
nations were not prepared for the camps, nor did they have any real
understanding of their nature or the policies and events that had
shaped them. Without such preparation and understanding, relief for
the victims was bound to prove difficult.

There were reasons for these deficiencies. Foremost among them
was that the camps revealed inhumanity beyond the contemporary
imagination. There was no way to prepare for the misery they
contained: the camps had to be witnessed to be believed; the extent
of the suffering had to be comprehended before the dimensions of
the relief effort could be conceived. The Allied governments had
considerable knowledge about the existence of an extensive network
of camps of all kinds throughout occupied Europe and Germany but
they did not have sufficient understanding of the camp system and the

mechanisms of genocide, nor did they know how, in these final stages of the war, those mechanisms were disintegrating.

In April–May 1945, conditions in the camps in Western Europe were worse than they had ever been and they were deteriorating daily. The British and American press dubbed the camps they liberated 'death camps', but they were not extermination camps. Those camps, built specifically to murder Jews, were all in the East, in Poland, and their closure and the evacuation of inmates from the path of the Red Army was in part the cause of the conditions the Western Allies uncovered. This was the breakdown of the system of slave labour and genocide, rather than its efficient operation. Evacuees were crammed into existing concentration, labour and prisoner-of-war camps. In the final weeks of the war, no one outside the camps knew exactly how many people they contained or what awful conditions prevailed inside.

We must also understand the Western Allies' lack of preparation for the liberation of the camps in the context of the closing weeks of a very long and costly war. Harsh as it might seem, defeating Germany as quickly as possible, rather than aiding its victims, was at this stage the Allies' main concern. The camps in the West were liberated over a very short period, and there was little time to respond to one before another was discovered. Those who bore responsibility for organising the relief effort – mainly military medical personnel trained to deal with battle casualties – had to undertake the task with no preparation and limited supplies. They had to move on very quickly from the shock of discovery to dealing with the practical realities of healing and survival of the victims. Those realities were indeed daunting. We must, therefore, judge the medical relief in the light of the immense task that they faced.

The liberation of the camps in the west occurred within a period of just four weeks. On 4 April 1945, the American 4th Armoured Division of the Third Army overran a camp at Ohrdruf in the north of Germany. In it, they found about 700 skeletal inmates, barely alive among more than 3000 unburied corpses. They were crammed into barracks and double-decker bunks, several to a bed. Most were suffering from running diarrhoea and covered in sores. Many were

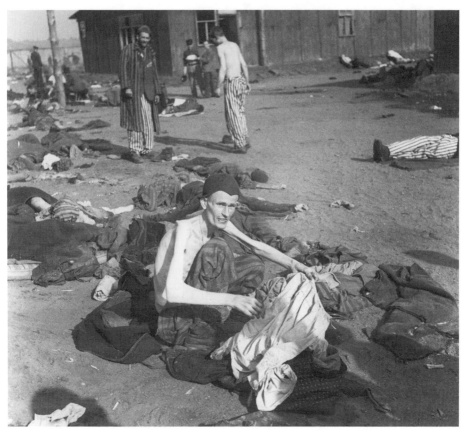

Up to 65,000 inmates of the Belsen concentration camp were found alive but most were in desperate need of medical assistance. (Image courtesy of bpk, Bildagentur für Kunst, Kultur und Geschicte, 30014487 bpk.)

clearly diseased. All were severely dehydrated since there was no water supply. There was no food, but the inmates displayed the effects of long-term malnutrition and starvation, some too weak to move.[2]

The shock of encountering this camp was soon overtaken by the discovery of more and larger camps in which the conditions were even worse, though at every stage of the liberation process no one could imagine worse. The overcrowding and filth meant that many inmates were suffering from festering wounds: deep ulcers, abscesses, gangrene and scabies were common. The larger camps were ridden with highly virulent disease: typhus, typhoid, tuberculosis, diphtheria, dysentery, and pneumonia. Of greatest concern was typhus, a highly infectious and lethal bacterial disease spread by lice. The military forces feared it because it posed a threat to liberating troops and to surrounding populations. The first impressions of the liberators frequently reflect the number and size of the lice that infected every inmate. In their accounts of recovery, survivors, who were often too sick to recall their treatment in any detail, do remember the sudden relief of being freed from their torment.[3]

Three days after the discovery of Ohrdruf, the Americans entered the larger complex of Dora-Nordhausen, where they found 3000 corpses and 2000 prisoners in similar conditions. They knew now that thousands of inmates were being evacuated in a disorganised way, in any direction that would avoid the Allied advance. Four days later, on 11 April, the American 4th and 6th Armored Divisions entered the main camp at the centre of these satellites. This was Buchenwald. Even though the majority of its 50,000 prisoners had been marched out only days earlier and the camp had effectively liberated itself, there was a remnant population of 21,000, including 700 children. A 'Little Camp' housed mainly Jews, Gypsies and recent evacuees in the most deplorable state. More than a thousand people were crammed into barracks built for 450. Many died where they lay and continued to do so for days after liberation.

The shock and challenge of dealing with Buchenwald was soon overtaken when, on 15 April, the 11th British Armoured Division entered the camp at Bergen-Belsen. They had more or less stumbled upon it when a German delegation had offered to surrender it, ostensibly because of a typhus outbreak. A truce and handover had to be arranged: this took three days. When the British troops entered, they found 60,000–65,000 inmates in two sites. There were 40,000–45,000 in the main camp, which became known as the 'horror camp', two-thirds of them women, and 500 children. Corpses were strewn everywhere. In the previous two weeks, 25,000–30,000 evacuees from other camps had been crammed into this already overcrowded area. In those two weeks an estimated 9000 had died. The food ration had become increasingly meagre and sporadic and had then ceased completely a week before the liberation. At the same time the camp authorities cut the water supply: people drank what they could from rain puddles contaminated with human excreta and corpses. There were probably about 10,000 dead when the British entered, but it was impossible to get an accurate figure because the number rose before any body count could be completed. As long as ten days after liberation, 500 people were dying every day: the daily death rate did not fall to below 100 until after the war in Europe was over. In those days before liberation, the dead lay among the living, who were too weak to remove the bodies. Many survivors could barely move themselves; they had no blankets and no clothing, just rags at best. The typhus cases – the number of which the Germans had severely underestimated – had not been isolated. Some barracks were so crowded that there was no room to lie down: excreta was 15 centimetres deep on the floor; the walls were caked with filth.[4]

Belsen was the first camp to be liberated before the Germans could begin to evacuate and shut it down – indeed, there was nowhere else that the Germans could send their victims – so conditions and overcrowding were worse there than in any other camp. For these reasons, Belsen has become the primary focus in assessing the medical relief of the camps. However, we should be wary of focusing too narrowly on Belsen. There were hundreds of smaller camps liberated over the next few days in which conditions were similar, though there were fewer dead. We should also not forget that the liberation of major camps was not yet over.

Dachau was the first Nazi concentration camp, built well before the war, so the Americans were not only well aware of its existence but they now had a greater sense of what they might find as they approached it. When the 45th Division liberated the camp on 29 April, there were approximately 70,000 inmates. By then the death rate was about 200 per day. Corpses lay unburied. The usual diseases raged, including typhus. Although the administration of the camp had not broken down to the extent it had in Belsen, supplies of food, water and electricity had ceased in the final days. Two days before liberation, however, a delegation from the International Committee of the Red Cross arrived at Dachau and persuaded the camp authorities to accept food. The day before that, more than 1700

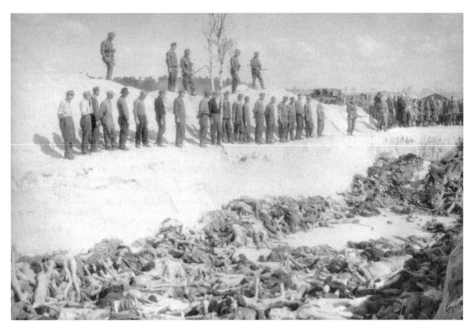

British soldiers force former SS guards of the Belsen concentration camp to attend a burial service at the open pit containing the corpses of their former prisoners, 16 April 1945. Despite efforts at medical care, up to 500 inmates continued to die every day for ten days after the camp was liberated. (AWM P03007.014)

people had arrived from the east, starving and weak from successive evacuations and death marches. About 2300 additional inmates sent from Buchenwald, however, never made it beyond the town's station. The Americans discovered their bodies still on the train: most had died from starvation and exposure but many had been shot or clubbed to death.

The last large camp to be liberated was Mauthausen in Austria. The Red Cross had convinced the commandant to accept food parcels from 22 April and had managed to extract some Western European deportees for repatriation, but gassings at the camp continued for another week.[5] With the co-operation of the local villagers and a last-minute surrender facilitated by the Red Cross, the American Third Army took the town and camp without a fight on 8 May. They found about 20,000 inmates. So brutal had the work regime been in this camp that some 3000 died in the days immediately following liberation. But that day, 8 May, was the day of the German surrender. For the victors, and certainly for the press and those on the home front keen to celebrate the peace, the liberation of the camps was complete. In reality, the real work of liberation – the medical relief – had only just begun.

Personnel from medical corps, casualty clearing stations and field hospitals were rushed in to relieve the suffering in the camps. Clearly they faced an immense task. So too did the civilian volunteers who soon followed them. They worked long hours under difficult conditions, seven days a week with little rest for weeks at a stretch. Their dedication is unquestioned. Often forced to learn as they went, they did the best they knew how. The organisation of the medical relief effort has proved controversial in the historical scholarship but criticism cannot be directed at the heroic efforts of these men and women.

The first issue in the historical controversy arises from the fact that the Western Allies were not prepared for the liberation of the camps. They could not have been fully prepared for the conditions they found, but the question remains whether they might not have been at least better prepared. The second issue arises from the fact that mistakes were made in the medical treatment of survivors and that a reasonably high proportion died after liberation: approximately a quarter of those alive at the liberation of Belsen died soon afterwards.[6] The historical scholarship on this issue divides into two schools: those who view the effort as essentially sound (that is, it was the best response possible under extremely difficult conditions); and those who see the response as flawed and in some ways inadequate, even taking account of the difficulties.[7]

The lack of any real preparation for the liberation of the camps means that the fundamental problem was a failure of political will that went back well before 1945. Western governments had early intelligence of German crimes against humanity and of the systematic murder of all Jews who fell under their control, but they did little to exploit it, let alone use it to make adequate preparations for dealing with the victims. The general public was informed by regular press reports about Nazi crimes and given the basic facts of the Final Solution. Before the close of 1942, the existence of extermination camps and the murder of an estimated two million Jewish civilians were reported in major Western newspapers. Exhibitions of smuggled photographs showing mass executions toured major cities in Britain and America in 1943: tens of thousands had attended.[8] The fact that Allied nations had the knowledge and the time to be better prepared for dealing with the victims of Nazi brutality, but failed to do so, indicates a general inability to comprehend how desperate these victims were, let alone to plan for the stream of refugees that would inevitably complicate the liberation of Europe and the defeat of Germany.

There was also more immediate and specific evidence of the camps. Nine months before the Western Allies uncovered Ohrdruf, the Soviets liberated the first concentration and extermination camps in the East.[9] A Western press delegation toured the extermination camp at Majdenek and reported on the gas chambers, mass graves and warehouses full of the belongings of an estimated one million victims. The British Foreign Office also had specific knowledge of Belsen. It knew that the head of the SS, Heinrich Himmler, had developed this Panzer training school into a camp for so-called 'prominent' and neutral Jews who could be bartered and exchanged for Germans living in Palestine. Such an exchange took place nine months before the liberation. Allied governments could, therefore, have better equipped their liberating forces with information about location of the camps and co-ordinated with aid organisations to assist survivors.

The international community also made little provision to deal with the problem of refugees and virtually none to cope with survivors of genocide. The Red Cross kept its knowledge of genocide hidden for fear that exposure would breach its neutrality and restrict its traditional role and access to prisoner-of-war camps. Its intervention in the concentration camps came very late – too late for so many who died in the last days. The United Nations came closest to recognising that civilian relief would be needed at war's end. In late 1943 it set up its Relief and Rehabilitation Administration (UNRRA) and planned 450 relief teams for the liberation. But, by 1945, it had managed to put together only eight teams and had not worked out a way to co-operate with the military forces.[10] No government, aid or military organisations had considered that victims of genocide might need special care: victims of the camps were to be treated as 'displaced persons' and counted in national groups so that they might be repatriated as soon as possible. Jews were not distinguished as a separate group, despite the obvious evidence of their greater suffering. There was little recognition that survivors might need long-term hospitalisation and medical treatment, that they might have no families or homes to which they could return or that it might be difficult to resettle unhealthy people.

The greatest failure in the liberation of the camps, therefore, was the Western Allies' failure to mount an effective response to a problem that was at least in part foreseeable. The result was that the relief of the camps was left to military medical units that were totally unprepared for the task. They were not equipped with knowledge, let alone with sufficient personnel, appropriate training, hospital facilities, medications, supply or transport.

In the first camps to be liberated medical units were not present and first aid was left to fighting units. As a result, most troops reacted with compassion and fed starving people emergency rations of chocolate or peanut butter and then army food that was too rich. Many survivors died immediately. The failure to prepare the liberators for what they might find in the camps meant that many were greatly shocked by the experience. This may explain why not everyone reacted with compassion, with some so revolted by the state of the camp inmates that they could not see them as human. One such British medical officer wrote after entering Neuengamme, a sub-camp of Sachsenhausen:

> One felt no pity for these people – only loathing [and] disgust . . . I toyed with the idea of pouring petrol around the place and setting the whole lot on fire. In my state of mind at the time the idea did not seem ridiculous: indeed it seemed to be the only possible solution.[11]

The senior medical personnel whose job it soon became to organise the relief deserve recognition for not being overwhelmed, as they so easily might have been, by the enormity of the task. The day after the liberation of Belsen, the Deputy Director of Medical Services of the British Second Army, Brigadier Glyn-Hughes, inspected the camp and determined that the 40,000 survivors in the 'horror camp' had to be removed from the atrocious conditions. Estimating that 70 per cent needed hospitalisation, he drew up a plan of triage, essentially to evacuate those likely to survive to a makeshift hospital set up in the German quarters.[12] But there were too many victims and not enough staff or resources. Three days after liberation, when the medical relief began, Glyn-Hughes had assembled a team of two Field Hygiene Units, a Casualty Clearing Station, a Light Field Ambulance and garrison troops. This amounted to only eight doctors, eight nurses and about 300 men. The selection of who lived and who died was almost arbitrary. The officer commanding the 11th Field Ambulance wrote:

> The MO [medical officer] went into each hut and marked on the forehead of each patient a cross to indicate to the bearers that this patient would be moved . . . [He] made no attempt to fix a diagnosis – all he did was to decide whether the patient had any chance of living if he or she were moved or what the chance of survival might be if the patient were left in the camp for another week. It was a heart-rending job and amounted to telling hundreds of poor wretches that they were being left to die.[13]

Removal to the hospital was severely slowed and limited, first by lack of transport and then by an insufficient number of hospital beds. At the hospital there were too few personnel to carry out the task of cleaning and delousing patients in what became known as the 'human laundry'. Patients were scrubbed of caked dirt, dusted with DDT and put into clean clothing and beds, twenty at a time.

Glyn-Hughes accepted, perhaps with a sense of resignation, that relief of the camp had been left to the army, but he also judged that only the Royal Army Medical Corps (RAMC) had the organisational skill to carry out the task. As a result, he was slow to call on outside help. He did call upon civilian emergency medical reinforcements from British Red Cross and St John's Ambulance but not on other civilian or International Red Cross organisations. Six British Red Cross detachments took a week to arrive from Holland and they proved much more successful in obtaining supplies from the civilian German population.[14] Ninety-one medical students from London arrived a further week after that. Four days later, more RAMC units were called in: two General Hospitals, a Field Ambulance, a Casualty Clearing Station and a Field Hygiene Section. German nurses were pressed into service – much to the horror of survivors – and eventually UN aid organisations relieved the first

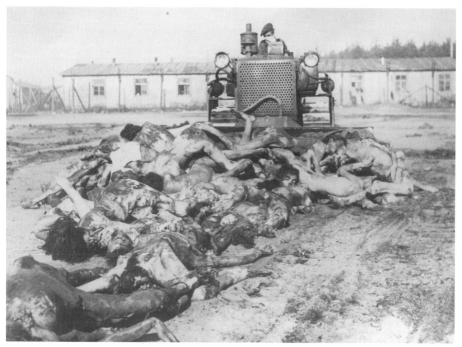

A British soldier uses a bulldozer to help bury the rotting corpses of prisoners at the Belsen concentration camp, 1945. The fear of disease and contamination made such measures imperative. (Image courtesy of bpk, Bildagentur für Kunst, Kultur und Geschicte, 30014490 bpk.)

medical teams. Evacuation of the horror camp took one month. By then, the first medical teams were exhausted and critical that more reinforcements had not been sent with more haste. As one medical student wrote on returning to Britain, the country was 'full of nurses rolling up face masks' who were needed in the camps.[15]

Even as the medical personnel increased, shortages remained acute. Two weeks after the relief began, one doctor wrote that all he had to treat open wounds, including deep ulceration to the bone, was aspirin and Dettol.[16] There was no provision of specialist medical care. Many survivors displayed the effects of psychological damage caused by starvation (famine psychosis) and severe emotional trauma, often sustained over several years. Such cases, some completely blank and unresponsive, others apathetic, deluded, deranged or violent, remained untreated because no one had considered that treatment for mental trauma would be a pressing need. Nutritional expertise in dealing with the psychological as well as physical effects of long-term starvation was also lacking. Medical staff had to learn by trial and error how and what to feed the survivors. Error was often fatal. The first meals were too rich and too large. The Bengal Famine Mixture – a concoction of dried milk, flour, sugar, salt and water which they hoped would re-hydrate the patients and be easily absorbed to give some energy – was not only so sweet that many could barely tolerate it but also far too rich for some. Attempts to administer hydration intravenously or to introduce the mixture via a stomach tube caused many survivors who knew of Nazi medical experimentation and execution in camp hospitals by lethal injection to recoil in terror. One medical student tolerated the death of five or six of his patients as a result of feeding by stomach tube before he finally refused to administer it.[17]

Lack of personnel also delayed the physical sanitation and evacuation of the camp. At first SS guards were forced to carry out the task of removal and burial of the dead by carrying or dragging the mass of corpses to huge pits. But this method proved too slow and fear of cholera meant that British troops were required to use bulldozers to move the bodies, which they did reluctantly. Even so,

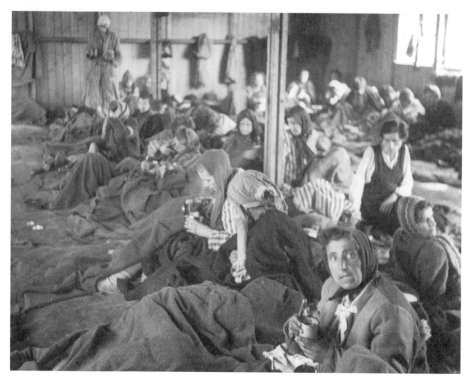

Former prisoners continued to live in squalid conditions in the camp huts at Belsen for weeks after liberation as the Allies struggled to deal with the scale of the human tragedy. (Image courtesy of bpk, Bildagentur für Kunst, Kultur und Geschicte, 30014934 bpk.)

the burial of bodies found at liberation took 11 days. The clearing, and then burning, of successive huts depended on the slow processes of the 'human laundry'. Three weeks after liberation, the war correspondent for the British *Daily Herald* reported that thousands of 'barely human' women remained in huts, even the best of which were 'encrusted with excreta' and offered nothing but bare boards to sleep on.[18]

Historian Paul Weindling is critical of Glyn-Hughes' traditional and methodical approach to sanitation and evacuation. He argues that it caused unnecessary delays as well as other problems that cost lives, the most serious of these being the failure to combat the typhus threat with modern, more rapid and effective means of spraying DDT. Delousing and dusting of each survivor in the 'human laundry' took two weeks to complete.[19] In one sense, this was a Herculean achievement, but the delay led to the infection of healthy survivors, many of whom were assisting in the relief effort. The effect can be seen in a spike in the death rate at Belsen after it had begun to drop following the liberation. By 26 April the rate had dropped to 343 per day, but a week later it increased again to 600.[20]

The RMAC's approach developed by Glyn-Hughes for Belsen was replicated in the subsequent relief of other camps and a similar spike in typhus-related deaths resulted. For example, at Sandbostel, which was liberated on 28 April, typhus infections doubled in three days from 9 May and increased by a further 25 per cent four days later. By then, the daily death rate had risen again to almost the rate it had been on liberation. The commanding medical officer nevertheless judged the control measures 'highly effective', since no British workers and 'only a few Germans' had contracted the disease.[21]

The British were slow to call on the United States Army Typhus Commission for assistance or to adopt their practices. This organisation had effectively stemmed the spread of typhus in Naples in 1943 and at the liberation sprayed high quantities of DDT throughout the camps. The US Army Surgeon General reported that all internees and all barracks at Dachau were being sprayed once a week. The result was that until three weeks after liberation cases of new infection ran at an average of 167 per day, but thereafter they dropped dramatically to 15 per day; death rates also declined and with no reported spike.[22]

Shortages, mainly in trained medical personnel but also in general labour, food, clothing and blankets, were the greatest problem reported in the relief of all camps. However, with experience, authorities seem to have resorted more rapidly and systematically to commandeering German supplies, impressing local labour, and employing German doctors and nurses. Two days after the liberation of Sandbostel, 200 German women arrived to help clean the camp and more arrived two days later, the additional aim being to expose as many German civilians as possible to the horrors of the camps.[23]

In many ways, the most important and difficult work in the liberation of the camps was achieved by medical personnel. They saved thousands of lives in spite of minimal preparation and with-

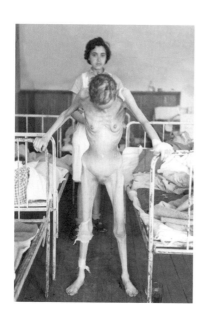

One month after liberation, a patient at the British hospital at the former concentration camp at Belsen still suffers the effects of prolonged starvation, disease and physical abuse, 16 May 1945.
(Image courtesy of bpk, Bildagentur für Kunst, Kultur und Geschicte, 30023150 bpk.)

out the resources to cope with the shocking nature and scale of the inhumanity uncovered in the camps. However, mistakes were made. The fundamental fault lay in a long-standing failure of political will. Had the Western Allies used the knowledge they had of the camps and made their relief part of their operational plan for the re-conquest of Europe, tens of thousands of lives could have been saved. These were the lives of those who died in the last few days before liberation. Many more might have survived had the liberators been armed with better knowledge and had they been backed by a co-ordinated plan to use all available resources to save the remaining victims of Nazi barbarity.

An Australian army doctor
– Bryan Gandevia

Simon C. Gandevia

In an interview published in the *Australian* in 1990 my father, Bryan Gandevia, recalled of his time in Korea: 'It was bitterly cold. Some of the fellows from WWII were complaining about aches in their old wounds, and we had many cases of frostbite.' The troops were ill-equipped in the early months: 'from a medical point of view, the supplies were a shambles'.[2]

I wrote this chapter for two reasons: firstly to present the observations of a young medical officer in the early months of Australia's involvement in the Korean War; secondly to sketch his later career and offer an assessment of it, in the process providing a broad context to the history award recently established in his memory.[3]

Bryan Gandevia was born into a medical family in Melbourne in April 1925. He completed his secondary education at Melbourne Grammar School, then studied medicine at the University of Melbourne, graduating in 1948. After completing his medical residency at the Royal Melbourne Hospital, in December 1949 he enlisted in the Royal Australian Army Medical Corps (RAAMC) with the rank of captain. Promoted to major, he served initially with

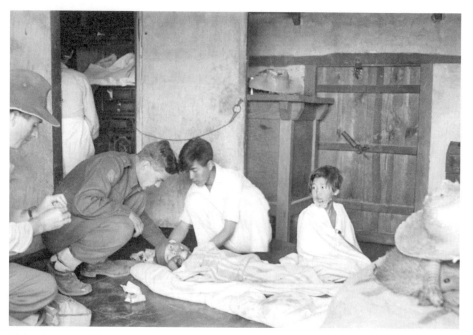

Major Bryan Gandevia, Regimental Medical Officer (RMO) with 3RAR, examines a Korean child with a facial gunshot wound from an American airstrike, October 1950, South Korea. (AWM P01472.019)

the British Commonwealth Occupation Force (BCOF) in Japan as a Regimental Medical Officer in the 3rd Battalion, Royal Australian Regiment (3RAR), before being deployed to Korea, where he served from September until late December 1950. While there he kept a diary and subsequently wrote and spoke about the effects of war and the harsh environment endured by the Australian soldiers.

It is worth considering why he enlisted so soon after becoming a doctor. He once mentioned to me that his enlistment was partly driven by having observed the effects the Second World War had had on the boys and families with whom he associated during his high-school years.

What did this 25-year-old captain, a comparative youngster in terms of both military and medical experience, think of his time in Korea? He noted frequently that the conditions were difficult and unpredictable. The temperature in mid-November was well below zero. For many of the men the snow was a novelty. The snow cover reached 45 centimetres, and this made evacuation of the wounded difficult: 'We had to use jeeps as ambulances', he wrote, 'which meant the wounded were exposed to the weather.' These observations recapitulated those in his formal medical report, published in 1951 not long after his return to Australia. His views had earlier been expressed when he was interviewed on location by Roy McCartney, war correspondent for the *Argus*. Although permission had been given for the interview to be conducted, the subsequent headline, 'Australians freeze in Korea: Medico tells . . .' led Prime Minister Robert Menzies to demand that they 'sack that bloody medical officer!'[4]

Report on medical and surgical aspects of the early Korean campaign

On his return to Melbourne, Bryan Gandevia prepared a paper for the *Medical Journal of Australia* which was published in August 1951.[5] He reported that in this period 'the Korean campaign presented a highly mobile warfare with intermittent battle in difficult terrain and rigorous climatic conditions'. Casualties resulted from enemy action, inclement weather and miscellaneous causes: the paper detailed casualties under those three categories. Under 'enemy action' the casualties from small-arms fire, mortars and hand grenades were described. 'Through and through' wounds were most common, with small entry and exit wounds. Heavy machine-gun wounds were often lethal. Casualties were less frequent than expected from mortar fire. Enemy stick grenades caused multiple 'peppering' wounds, rarely more than an inch deep. Few casualties resulted from anti-tank and anti-personnel mines, or aerial activity. The field experience was largely of gunshot wounds, moderate shrapnel wounds and compound fractures. Major thoraco-abdominal trauma was 'in the minority'.

Treatment at the regimental aid post (RAP) first consisted of 'no more than a minimum of first aid'. Morphine was given by the stretcher-bearers. 'Tea or coffee was usually provided by the padre' – a form of fluid replacement that has largely been dispensed with in modern warfare. Field and shell dressings, along with temporary splints, were applied and penicillin in oil was given routinely.

The next, and possibly most interesting, section of the paper dealt with casualties resulting from exposure to the cold, particularly frostbite. Gandevia noted the difficulty of distinguishing this condition from trench foot: the latter condition is associated with immersion in cool but not necessarily freezing temperatures; frostbite rarely affected the face and hands, so that factors other than the cold alone appeared to cause the preponderance of frostbite in the feet. He argued that although the American winter ('snowpac') boots were waterproof (rubber to the ankle and leather to mid-calf), 'eventually the accumulation of sweat began to freeze'. Unfortunately, circumstances commonly made it impossible for the troops to change socks and insoles daily as ordered.[6]

Gandevia provided a detailed listing of signs and symptoms drawn from his experience of approximately 100 cases of varying severity of frostbite. The key features were painful burning in the soles and balls of the feet, and wet feet, soggy with patches of white wrinkled skin. Subsequently, the feet became pinkish-blue and soft subcutaneous tissues swelled with pitting oedema. There were areas of ulceration, skin discolouration and blistering. Heat perception was always impaired but increased sensitivity was rare.

Frostbite sufferers with major skin changes were evacuated as quickly as possible. Treatment consisted of rest, elevation and foot hygiene, together with active treatment by massage with Vaseline, lanolin or oily brushless shaving cream. The advantage of the shaving cream was that it was easily obtained and remained semi-fluid in the low temperatures. No gangrene or secondary infections occurred in those not evacuated. The cold exacerbated a number of other conditions; these included fibrositis or myositis, for which injection of local anaesthetic with adrenaline was effective. Pain in the joints and the sites of old injuries or recent wounds was often severe. Pyelitis and bronchitis, but rarely pneumonia, were encountered. Cold limited the administration of penicillin. Penicillin in oil was carried in the pocket or kept in a bunk. The problem with the more rapidly acting crystalline penicillin was the need to thaw distilled water in order to inject the drug.

Among the miscellaneous causes of casualties were accidental wounds. They were 'not uncommon', but no data were included. Traffic accidents were common, but with few casualties. Dental treatment

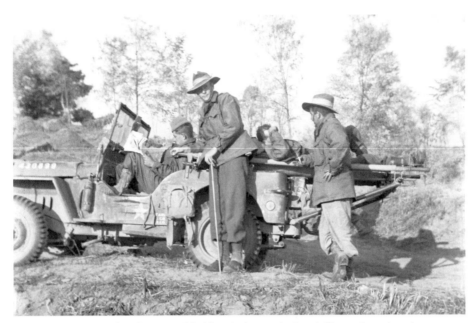

In the absence of field ambulances in South Korea, American jeeps were adapted to carry uncovered stretchers. Standing in front of the jeep is Captain Edward Manchester, a medical officer, and an unnamed stretcher bearer, November 1950. (AWM P01472.010)

was difficult to arrange for those with broken dentures. There were occasional cases of inner and outer ear infections. Gastroenteritis occurred frequently and, given the primitive sanitation, 'the importance of strict hygiene measures could not be over-emphasized'.

The inoculation program against typhoid, typhus, cholera and tetanus was compulsory and effective. Influenza vaccine and inoculation against Japanese B encephalitis had also been given to the majority of troops. Again, no cases of these diseases occurred.

In the final section of his paper Gandevia discussed some of the practical difficulties associated with the evacuation of casualties. Travelling on open jeeps fitted with stretchers exposed the wounded troops to the cold, especially at night, and so the assistance of the Americans' enclosed and centrally heated ambulances was sometimes requested. 'The combination of distance, difficult roads, heavy traffic and consequent slow speed introduced a serious time factor.' The distribution of available medical personnel among the companies is described. Four stretcher-bearers were allocated.[7] Difficulties were experienced owing to the dynamic nature of the conflict. A shuttle

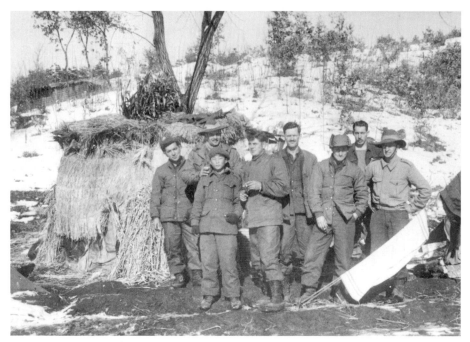

RMO Major Bryan Gandevia (second from left, at rear) with a group of fellow Australians and a South Korean boy near the 3RAR tent lines during the winter of 1950. Gandevia described the harsh effects of winter on the health of Australian soldiers fighting in Korea. (AWM P01472.011.)

service was set up between the regimental aid post and the field ambulance, with a final relay to the American services. Despite the 'array of difficulties' only three casualties reaching the regimental aid post died before being admitted to hospital. One of these died from multiple abdominal wounds, one from a compound fracture of the thigh, and one from an extensive upper abdominal wound.

The second part of the article in the *Medical Journal of Australia* was written by Lieutenant Colonel Hughes and Major Webb, and it dealt with the treatment of open wounds among British Commonwealth casualties.[8] It described the treatment of more than 300 open-wound casualties who had been evacuated from the front line via American forward hospitals and had reached the main base within five days of originally being wounded.

Gandevia was invited to give a talk about his experiences of the early parts of the Korean campaign to the Victorian Branch of the British Medical Association on 20 November 1951. He spoke of the extraordinary apathy of the Australian people and the indifference they showed to the war in Korea at the time, pointing out that he had even been asked whether the Australians had suffered any serious casualties.[9]

In hindsight, like many exposed to the trauma of conflict, Gandevia was impressed by the 'fantastic, sardonic, dry and pithy humour' of the soldiers. He recalled a young orderly, frightened by the thought that one of the bullets whizzing by might hit him, whose sergeant quipped, 'it's not the one with your name on it you need to worry about, it's the one marked to whom it may concern'.[10]

Medical Career after Korea

After his Korean service, Bryan Gandevia returned to the Royal Melbourne Hospital, where he worked as a Fellow in Industrial Medicine in the Department of Medicine. He also held an appointment in the Department of Anatomical Pathology at the University of Melbourne. His university appointment allowed him to develop an interest in pulmonary pathophysiology. In 1953 he obtained his Doctorate in Medicine from the university, and was admitted to the Royal Australasian College of Physicians (RACP). Thereafter, his main clinical and research work focused on respiratory medicine. To obtain further training, from 1954 to 1957, he worked in respiratory medicine in London at the Royal Brompton Hospital and the Royal Postgraduate Medical School. At the time, these were leading clinical and academic units in their field.

In 1963 Gandevia moved to Sydney to take up positions in the newly established medical school of the University of New South Wales. He was appointed Associate Professor of Medicine and the Inaugural Chairman of the Department of Respiratory Medicine at the Prince Henry and Prince of Wales Hospitals. He established clinical and research services and set up laboratories from which much of his major work derived. He held these positions until 1985, when he retired to a part-time practice in Randwick in Sydney. When work and other commitments allowed, he lived in a city apartment or at Mt Victoria in the Blue Mountains.[11]

Gandevia's research interests were in epidemiology and

occupational lung disease. He established a large mobile research laboratory which could screen industrial populations at their worksites. At the time, and perhaps even now, this was an advanced enterprise. The laboratory provided the full suite of simple and complex lung function tests, with the aim being to obtain an accurate snapshot of the respiratory health of workers exposed to potentially deleterious airborne particles. These exposures include asbestos, cotton and wheat dust, coal and others. The aim was to understand pathological changes induced by exposure and, ultimately, to influence industries to change practices to protect employees.

Over this period, he recruited several key staff, the most distinguished of whom was Associate Professor John Colebatch, whose pioneering work on the mechanical behaviour of the lung found direct application in the epidemiological survey work. Colebatch followed Gandevia as head of department. Gandevia also contributed to the training of a number of leading physicians, physiologists and epidemiologists, including Dr Charles Mitchell, Dr Ian Greaves, Dr Graham Hall, Dr Margaret Smith and Dr Bill Finucane, to name but a few. His final PhD student was Dr David McKenzie, who later became head of the Department of Respiratory Medicine after it had been led by Professor Colebatch.[12] Gandevia's research and clinical practice resulted in many publications in respiratory, epidemiological, and general clinical journals. Throughout this period, however, he had pursued an equally active career as a medical and social historian.

Career in history

Since his days as a medical student, Bryan Gandevia was deeply interested in medical history in its broadest form. On his return to Melbourne from London, he contributed to the vibrant Victorian branch of the British Medical Association which had a large collection of historical works and a museum. He published important aids directed in part to helping others in the task of historical research. The first of these was *An Annotated Bibliography of the History of Medicine in Australia*, published by the Australian Medical Association in 1956.[13]

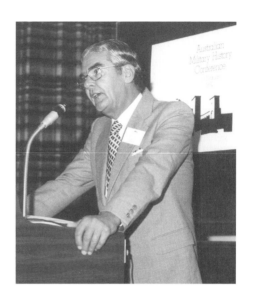

Professor Bryan Gandevia
speaking at the inaugural
Australian War Memorial Military
History Conference, February 1982.
(Image courtesy of Simon Gandevia,
from Bryan Gandevia papers.)

After moving to Sydney, he immediately became a driving member of the RACP Library Committee, of which he was Chairman from 1983 to 1994. Over a long period the previous Chairman, Sir Edward Ford, Gandevia and others helped to transform the library's rather disparate and dilapidated collection to a national resource library with a special interest in Australasian medical history. Gandevia's 'foresight and enthusiastic zeal' in this task was formally recognised.[14] At times, he needed to persuade the College Council to direct monies and resources to the task. Where the collection was weak, he made many donations from his personal library.

In 1984 he published (with Alison Holster, the RACP librarian, and Sheila Simpson, a retired medical librarian) a revised bibliography, titled *Annotated Bibliography of the History of Medicine and Health in Australia*.[15] This major work reflected the decision 'to broaden the scope to include aspects of social history impinging upon health and disease', as spelled out in the Introduction. More than 2700 items were catalogued. The strong relationship between Gandevia and Ford contributed to the donation of Ford's extraordinary collections to the RACP library, contributing to it being a major national and even international resource in some areas.

With the rise in importance of the collection, a joint Bicentennial project involving the RACP and the Commonwealth Department of Community Services and Health was established to publish a catalogue of all books and publications in medicine and health in Australia. The resulting four-volume *Bibliography of Australian Medicine and Health Services* was published in 1988.[16]

Not content with a role in these projects, Gandevia contributed frequently to the *Australian Dictionary of Biography* and acquired his own national and international reputation in the history of medicine, with many scholarly publications.

Further insight into his views about history, and in particular the history of medicine, can be derived from looking at one of his important works, *Tears often shed: child health and welfare in Australia from 1788*.[17] Far more than a simple history of Australian paediatrics, this was an attempt to combine history and medicine to explore not only how the practice of child health developed in Australia, but how the colony in Sydney began and evolved. For example, Gandevia wanted to glean as much as possible about the weights and heights of those living in the various penal colonies, along with information about their diseases and diets, their backgrounds and living conditions. He was striving to understand the interactive web that underpins a society and its interaction with the environment.

The book's preface stated its aim: to 'examine the medical aspects against the social and environmental background, to note the influence of social and environmental change on disease and health, and to consider the impact of medical developments on society and its attitudes'. Gandevia hoped that the work would 'help to break down the disciplinary barriers which are separated by social and medical history'. Interestingly, he frequently used quotations of Australian poetry to illustrate contemporary issues and social views. His preference for poetry rather than newspaper reports, the conventional technique used in social history, reflected his view that 'poets for the most part expressed themselves better than journalists, and usually after more profound thought'.[18] He followed this major work with a small volume intended for younger readers, *Life in the First Settlement at Sydney Cove*.[19]

Gandevia's role at the Australian War Memorial

In 1967, in part because of his service in Korea and his academic credentials in history, Gandevia was appointed a Trustee and later a Council member of the Australian War Memorial. Over the following sixteen years serving on the Board of Trustees and Council of the Memorial, he made a substantial contribution to the institution and helped to shape its future directions, most notably through changes designed to develop military historical research and publication. In 1976 he promoted the establishment of a research grants scheme which made awards in particular to younger researchers who, it was thought, might take a broader view of history than that offered by the official war historians. Gandevia also hoped the Memorial would foster the exchange of ideas through the establishment of a journal and regular military history conferences.[20]

Not all publication proposals were acceptable to the Memorial, however. On one notable occasion, Gandevia's response to a request by then Prime Minister Gough Whitlam led to a 'hell of a row'. Whitlam had wanted the Memorial to publish a collection of irreverent and bawdy songs by Second World War airmen. As Gandevia put it, 'the book would be published over my dead body', and indeed, the publication did not go ahead.[21] This may have motivated Whitlam to attempt to block Gandevia's reappointment to the Memorial's Council in 1975, although his appointment was reconfirmed by the Fraser government the following year.

Bryan Gandevia was subsequently awarded an Order of Australia for his work with the Australian War Memorial. He died in September 2006. Immediately after returning to Australia, Gandevia had donated his diary, papers and photographs relevant to his service in Korea to the Australian War Memorial; since his death, some of his other papers have been donated to the Mitchell Library.[22] The legacy of his contributions to medicine, history and the Australian War Memorial will undoubtedly be remembered and perpetuated through the history prize in his name.

Diggers and a 'dose of the clap': the problem of sexually transmitted infections among Australian soldiers in Vietnam

David Bradford [1]

'Venereal diseases have been a major cause of lost soldier strength in the wars of the 20th Century.'[2] (United States Army official history)

Introduction

Venereal diseases (VD), or sexually transmitted infections (STI), as they are now called, have always posed a threat to the health and well-being of soldiers serving in stressful wartime situations away from home. Australian defence forces have a reasonable record of paying attention to the sexual health of their servicemen and women, largely because of the pioneering work undertaken during the First World War by a courageous New Zealand woman, Ettie Rout (1877–1936).[3] STIs were a notable problem during the Vietnam conflict in that rates of infection remained high throughout the years of Australia's commitment despite the best efforts of successive Directors of Medical Services to control their incidence. Although they tended to cause less manpower wastage than in previous wars, owing to the availability of effective antibiotics and the ability of medical personnel to treat most infections in the field, STIs added considerably to the general discomfort and stress for the average soldier 'in country' and were an ever-present topic of uneasy conversation among officers and men alike. In addition, senior officers were well aware that STIs had the potential to create political problems should the high rates among the troops in Vietnam become widely known in the general Australian community.

The STI problem
The physical effects of the STIs encountered during the Vietnam War ranged from mild to severe, but the psychological effects on soldiers were sometimes more important. As human immunodeficiency virus (HIV) infection did not appear until the early 1980s, there was no fatal and untreatable STI in Vietnam or Southeast Asia during the 1960s and early 1970s. In previous wars, right up until the Malayan Emergency, almost all soldiers with STIs were treated in hospital, causing considerable manpower wastage. [4] In Vietnam most STIs could be managed on an outpatient basis, but in the period January 1967 to June 1968, hospital admissions for STIs ranged from 76 to 116 per six-month period. By July–December 1969, STI hospital admissions were down to only 28.[5] Modern medicine has greatly reduced time out of action caused by STIs and the number of unpleasant complications from STIs, but it has *not* reduced the rate of infection.

During the Vietnam conflict STI rates (recorded as a total of hospital admissions and outpatient cases per 1000 service personnel per year) were consistently two to four times higher than the admission rates for both malaria and all other fevers, and those for injuries (both war injuries and others).[6] The highest STI rate occurred in October 1966 (943 cases per 1000 soldiers per year); the lowest STI rate came in May 1969, at 128 per 1000 per year.[7] It is perhaps notable that the township of Vung Tau with its bars and brothels was out of bounds to all Australian forces for the first few months of 1969 because of the fear of a second Tet Offensive.

During 1967–68 the STI rate remained fairly consistently high (for example, an average of 478 cases per 1000 soldiers per year throughout 1967). There was a noticeable drop in February 1968 to 170 cases per 1000 per year.[8] In his Vietnam official history volume, *Medicine at War*, Brendan O'Keefe remarks:

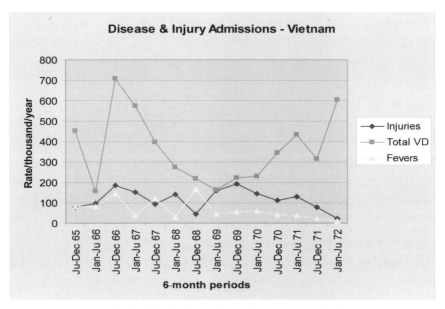

Disease & Injury Admissions - Vietnam

**Hospital admissions for disease and injury
among Australian soldiers in South Vietnam,
July 1965 to July 1972**

Total VD = Hospital admissions plus outpatient diagnoses
Fevers = Malaria plus other specific and non-specific fevers
Injuries = Battle injuries plus all other injuries requiring admission

Compiled by David Bradford from data in Brendan G. O'Keefe,
*Medicine at War: Medical aspects of Australia's involvement in
Southeast Asia 1950-1972*, 1994, Allen & Unwin in
association with the Australian War Memorial,
Sydney, 1994, Appendix C.

In the short term, the only noteworthy, though regrettably short-lived drop in the VD rate was brought about by the Tet Offensive. Vung Tau with its dubious attractions remained out of bounds during the offensive and the soldiers themselves were perhaps more fully occupied with the business of survival.[9]

Gavin Hart's work

Captain Gavin Hart was a medical officer at the 1st Australian Field Hospital (1AFH) at Vung Tau during 1970. As he had a major interest in STIs, he used his time there to conduct a series of surveys that examined the sexual behaviour and psychological characteristics of Australian soldiers during their time in Vietnam. These studies, which formed the basis of his MD thesis at the University of Adelaide, were subsequently published in the *British Journal of Venereal Diseases*.[10] His findings, from a questionnaire of 376 soldiers of the rank of sergeant or below returning to Australia after their tour of duty, included the following results:

- They were young, with more than 85 per cent less than 26 years old.

- Sexual experience: only 1.6 per cent had never had sex at all (1 per cent had sex for the first time in South Vietnam).

- Sex in Vietnam: 65.5 per cent had sex in Vietnam, which means that just over a third of the men actually abstained from sex in Vietnam.

- 'Rest and recreation' leave (R&R) in a Southeast Asian city: by 1970, only 36 per cent took their R&R in a Southeast Asian city; but of those who did, 94.5 per cent had sex there. (NB: In 1970, 64 per cent had their 'R&R' in Sydney.)

- Only 22.5 per cent of soldiers used condoms (15 per cent of single men; 39.5 per cent of married men).

- 29 per cent reported that they were 'influenced into having sexual intercourse by alcohol'.

- Of those exposed through sexual intercourse, 27 per cent contracted an STI.

- 10.5 per cent of those exposed had an STI more than once.

- When asked why they had abstained from sex, the abstainers responded:
  - Desire to be faithful (married men) to a wife at home – 67 per cent. (NB: Having a steady girlfriend or a fiancée back home did not seem to have the same influence on fidelity as being married.)
  - Fear of VD –10 per cent
  - Lack of opportunity – 8 per cent.

Perhaps Hart's most notable finding was that 'no soldier who used a condom on all occasions acquired VD'. He thus confirmed that condoms are effective, something that Ettie Rout had claimed during the First World War.

My experience as a regimental medical officer

I arrived in Vietnam in May 1967 and returned to Australia in May 1968. I was Regimental Medical Officer (RMO) for 4 Field Regiment, Royal Australian Artillery – 'a gunners' doctor'.[11] I spent most of my 12 months at Nui Dat where the 1st Australian Task Force (1ATF) was located. I was assigned to the Headquarters Battery of 4 Fd Regt and travelled with the battery whenever it moved to establish a fire support base (FSB) in the field on active operations. I took part in several operations including 'Paddington', 'Ballarat', 'Kenmore', 'Ainslie', 'Santa Fe', 'Duntroon' and 'Coburg'.

During my time Nui Dat was home to the task force headquarters, two (later three) infantry battalions, the artillery regiment, a cavalry squadron (with later a tank squadron), the Special Air Service Regiment (SASR), engineers and other supports, an airfield and several helicopter pads, and a forward detachment of Vung Tau's 8 Field Ambulance (later to become a full field ambulance when the Vung Tau Hospital was upgraded to 1AFH). In addition, there was

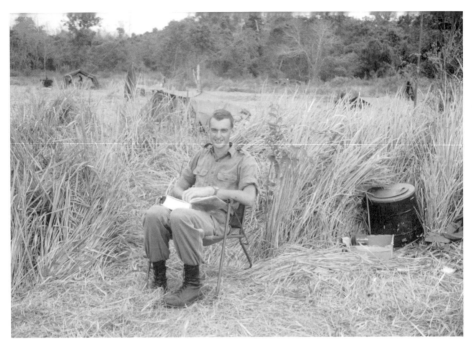

Captain David Bradford, medical officer with 4 Field Regiment, reading a medical textbook next to a spare latrine at a fire support base during Operation Duntroon, South Vietnam, January 1968. (Image courtesy of David Bradford.)

a chapel and a cricket pitch. There were four doctors at Nui Dat in 1967, one with each of the two battalions, one at the Forward Detachment of 8 Field Ambulance and myself.

In general, all soldiers at Nui Dat spent 12 months there. The only leave during that time was five days' 'rest and convalescence' leave (R&C) in Vung Tau (30 kilometres away) and five days' R&R leave in a Southeast Asian city (or, increasingly, from November 1967 onwards, in Sydney). Nui Dat was an unusual environment. Soldiers were confined to their units there or travelled with them on patrol or on operations outside the base for 50 of their 52-week period of service in Vietnam.

There were no women at 1ATF, therefore Australian troops in Nui Dat had very little contact with women for 12 months. Their only possible contacts were with:

- Australian Army or New Zealand Army nurses (four only in 1967) in the hospital at Vung Tau.
- Red Cross workers (one or two only) at Vung Tau.

- Vietnamese women and girls in nearby Vietnamese villages or the countryside (it was quite uncommon for most soldiers at Nui Dat to meet these).
- Women met on R&R or R&C leave (usually bar girls).
- Visiting Australian women in concert entertainment groups (but only on stage).

Australian soldiers at Nui Dat were generally young, fit and healthy. However, they had no social outlets, they were subject to constant strain and stress, from time to time their lives were in danger and, because prostitution was rife in Vietnam and other Southeast Asian cities, any opportunities for the men to mix with women who were not prostitutes while on leave were severely restricted.

Being an RMO at Nui Dat was very like being a general practitioner, except that RMOs were on duty 24 hours a day, seven days a week; conducted a regular morning surgery ('sick parade'); had an all-male youthful clientele (the average age for the men of the regiment was about 25); and their patients usually had some barrier to overcome before being able to attend a sick parade, in that they required permission from their immediate superior, or at least from their battery medic.

Among most officers there was a climate of opinion that a soldier needed to be really sick or injured before attending sick parade. The 2IC of 4 Field Regiment was heard to remark on many occasions in my hearing: 'You can tell how good an RMO is by the size of his sick parade … a good RMO has the smallest sick parade possible.' Doubtless he thought I failed dismally on this criterion. Nevertheless, soldiers did attend sick parade, and usually for respiratory problems: colds, coughs and chest infections, skin conditions (especially fungal and foot problems), gastric upsets and dysentery, injuries (there was a wide range of these, but actual war wounds and injuries were relatively uncommon among the gunners), and tropical conditions such as fevers (including malaria), ear infections and ulcers. In addition, there were symptoms resulting from the effects of alcohol and the full range of STIs. Underlying psychological problems frequently masqueraded as something physical, as a physical symptom was often the only way a distressed soldier could get to attend sick parade.

STIs in Vietnam

The particular STIs encountered in Vietnam included the following (in order of frequency):

- Gonorrhoea (urethral discharge and painful urination), more commonly know as 'the clap'.
- NSU (non-specific urethritis): a milder urethral discharge than gonorrhoea.
- Chancroid (soft sore): a tropical STI, which caused genital ulcers.
- Syphilis (genital ulceration and generalised disease), commonly called 'the pox'.
- Genital herpes (genital blisters and sores)
- Genital warts (warty lesions on the genitalia)
- Crabs (pubic lice) and scabies (generalised itch, lumps on penis and scrotum).
- Rarer tropical STIs that caused genital ulceration (for example, LGV (lymphogranuloma venereum) and donovanosis).

There were some problems associated with STIs specific to Vietnam. First, accurate diagnosis was often difficult under field conditions – RMOs had access to a microscope for examining smears but results of confirmatory tests took some time to come back from Vung Tau. Second, we did encounter resistance to antibiotics – about 10 per cent of cases of gonorrhoea were resistant to standard treatment with penicillin during Australia's years in Vietnam.[12] Third, NSU (which we now know was mostly due to chlamydia) was difficult to treat as it required at least seven days of tetracycline to clear. The dosage was awkward – two capsules, four times daily – and the capsules tended to get soggy in the hot humid climate.

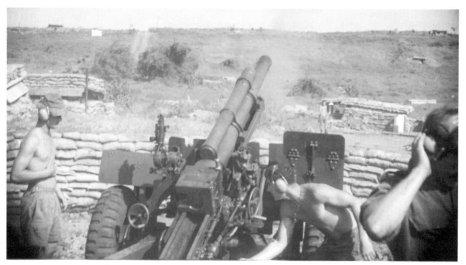

Gunners of 4 Field Regiment carrying out a fire mission at the Horseshoe base, Phuoc Tuy province, South Vietnam, 1967. (Image courtesy of David Bradford.)

A diagnosis of syphilis needed daily penicillin injections for seven to ten days. While these could be administered in the field or at Nui Dat, sometimes hospitalisation was required to ensure that the course of treatment was completed.

Physical complications of STIs were fairly uncommon, but when they did occur hospitalisation became essential. Such complications were persistent urethral symptoms, usually due to incomplete courses of treatment; epididymo-orchitis (swollen, painful testis); and disseminated infections (joint involvement, skin rashes, fever, and systemic symptoms).

Psychological complications were more subtle and varied, but in my experience were common. These included guilt and low self-esteem (probably the most common outcomes), a sense of shame, resort to alcohol, depression, anxiety (especially as 'return to Australia' [RTA] approached), a belief that cure was impossible, and sometimes even panic attacks.

There were some commonly held views back then (and the same can still be heard even today) which militated against good control of STIs. These included the belief that STIs were a trivial nuisance, that patients with STIs were a feckless bunch, and that a quick antibiotic shot or script was all that was required. In fact, good medical management of STIs is fundamentally important because sympathy and empathy win patient confidence and compliance with treatment. Patient co-operation is essential if adequate contact tracing is to be achieved, and if public health aspects are to be successfully addressed. Recognition and treatment of the psychological consequences of STIs are an essential part of best practice.

In November 1967 I undertook a three-week posting to Saigon, during which I visited American medical units and hospitals within the area and conducted morning sick parade for Australian soldiers posted at the Free World Military HQ in the city. I formed the impression that STIs were even more of a problem for soldiers working in the capital than at Nui Dat.

Prevention of STIs

As far as the Army Medical Corps in Vietnam was concerned, the dice were heavily stacked against achieving any sort of control of the STI problem. Many of the most important causative factors were beyond our control: for example, the 'caged in' existence at Nui Dat, the stressful environment, youthful hormones with no social outlets, and widespread prostitution (in particular, the easy availability of cheap sex workers in Vung Tau). In addition, the culture of R&R and R&C leave actually promoted risk-taking, with commercial interests ensuring that a soldier's every need was met when he was on leave.

During 1967 Lieutenant Colonel Meyer, CO of 8 Field Ambulance, continued a system of free medical examinations and treatment for prostitutes working in bars and brothels in Vung Tau, and instituted a system of ID cards for all 'bar girls', issuing each with a clinical card. Establishments that failed to comply with these measures were placed off-limits, and the army provosts were expected to enforce these restrictions. In practice, this proved impractical given the small number of available provosts, and so the STI rate remained largely unaffected.[13]

Back at Nui Dat, the RMOs did what they could to reduce the rates of STIs. We gave numerous lectures to all ranks in an attempt to raise awareness and our medics did the same. Our major message was 'try to abstain from sex until you get back home'. We promoted the use of condoms and at 4 Field Regiment standing orders required that all soldiers (from the CO down) had to attend the regimental aid post before going on leave to obtain a packet of a dozen condoms. We gave warnings about the effects of alcohol on lowering inhibitions, and we all adopted a non-punitive approach to STIs, encouraging soldiers to get checked after episodes of unprotected sex. An RTA check-up was compulsory before a soldier could leave for home; this included a full physical examination and a blood test for syphilis.

Despite such measures, STIs remained a constant problem throughout the whole period of Australia's involvement in Vietnam. Gavin Hart has summed it up excellently:

> The venereal disease impact in this situation was . . . a consequence of the environment. The environmental stress of a war situation produced behaviour patterns which many participants would not otherwise experience. Sexual behaviour normally encountered in a minority group becomes the experience of the majority of the population.[14]

Effects of alcohol

Alcohol has both physical and mental effects. Physical effects can result from acute intoxication or alcohol poisoning. Alcohol can irritate the gastric lining, resulting in gastritis, gastro-intestinal bleeding, and (rarely) acute ulceration with perforation of the stomach or duodenal wall. Its chronic effects on the liver are well known and can result in cirrhosis of the liver and eventual liver failure. The heart and both the central and peripheral nervous systems can also be damaged by chronic alcohol abuse.

The mental effects of alcohol can be both acute and chronic. In Vietnam we were most concerned with the acute effects of binge drinking, which could result in lowered inhibitions and risk-taking, temporary but significant personality changes (for example, impulsive behaviour and aggression), and acute behavioural changes, leading to a spectrum of acts of indiscipline (such as minor acts of omission, self-harm, and commission of serious acts of disobedience resulting in harm to fellow soldiers).

I hope my comments on this subject are not coloured by the fact that I was a teetotaler during my time in Vietnam. It seemed to me at that time, however, that Australian military forces had a definite alcohol tradition. It was common to hear remarks like 'a soldier ought to be able to handle his drink', '*real* men know how to drink well', and 'we work hard and we play hard'. While it was certainly not the case in 4 Field Regiment, many officers (at all levels) maintained a climate where alcohol abuse was not only common but actually encouraged.

Almost inevitably, RMOs frequently became involved where there were episodes of indiscipline involving alcohol. Our major underlying concern was the ready availability of firearms, everywhere and at all times, at the base at Nui Dat and the FSBs out in the field. We were consulted when soldiers were drunk on duty ('Is this gunner drunk, doc?'); when there were 'accidents' with weapons (some accidental loss of life certainly occurred at Nui Dat); and where there were instances of self-harm (in particular, self-inflicted injuries, threatening or violent behaviour, or when actual physical harm to others had occurred). In addition, excessive use of alcohol sometimes led to episodes of psychological distress and breakdown (such as uncontrolled crying, withdrawal from others, numbness, bizarre behaviour) and episodes of clinical depression.

'Winning hearts and minds' and the MEDCAP (Medical Civil Aid Program)

Each RMO was allocated a couple of villages near Nui Dat where he would make regular weekly or fortnightly visits in order to hold a clinic for the local villagers. In addition, during the course of a military operation, an RMO located at a temporary FSB might be directed to make a special visit to provide a clinic in a nearby village in an attempt to compensate for the inconvenience caused by the operation. The RMO would be accompanied by a couple of medics, an interpreter from the South Vietnamese forces (ARVN), and three or more soldiers from the regiment to provide protection ('shot guns').

There were advantages and disadvantages to a MEDCAP. The advantages were that it was a good chance to meet the people and to provide some medical service for villagers. It was possible to make some appropriate referrals for tuberculosis, injuries or serious illness. And the program may have fostered some goodwill.

On the down side, the operation of the program was patchy and inconsistent and always contingent on operational necessity. Overall, it was very much a 'band-aid' approach, carried out under less than ideal circumstances. There was very good evidence that the drugs being given out were frequently diverted to the Viet Cong. And although no Australian medical personnel ever came to any harm on a MEDCAP mission, there was potential danger for any medico conducting a clinic in a potentially hostile village with only a small handful of soldiers to protect him. As I describe in my book, the only occasion on which I actually felt afraid during my year in Vietnam was during a MEDCAP clinic in a village I had never visited before.[15]

Conclusion

The experience of the Australian Army in Vietnam showed that STIs continued to be a problem for the troops, even though they did not result in the manpower wastage seen in earlier conflicts. The incidence of STIs was just one of the harmful effects associated with excessive use of alcohol. Commanders of any military force on active service in a war zone must always take account of the needs of their troops, whether these pertain to mental health, sexual health, or recreation. In particular, officers have a duty to promote the responsible and rational use of alcohol, and this is something that must proceed from the top down.

Surgery under fire: civilian surgical teams in Vietnam

Elizabeth Stewart[1]

On 4 January 1967 Australian nursing sister Dorothy Angell wrote home to her parents from Bien Hoa at the start of her Vietnam tour of duty:

> Dearest Mum & Dad,
> Well here I am back from the first day's work; tired, filthy but happy. The work is really cut out for us out here, but even though today was a bit of a shambles I think everyone is really going to work well together.[2]

Eleven days later Sister Angell wrote again and it was clear that reality had set in:

> Dearest family,
> We are still flat out at the hospital and there has not been one night when we haven't been called out to attend an emergency . . . Last Friday night they had to operate on a woman with a <u>live</u> shell embedded in her stomach, then

last night we had a 3 year old brought in with half its brain hanging out from a grenade explosion. It's when you see the children that you get upset.[3]

Dorothy Angell was one of many nurses from hospitals all over Australia who volunteered to work as part of a civilian surgical team in South Vietnam during its bitter and protracted war against the North. Angell was from Melbourne's Alfred Hospital, one of several teaching hospitals to send teams, the first in October 1964, and the last in late 1972. Australian teams were sent initially to Long Xuyen, then to Bien Hoa, Vung Tau and finally Ba Ria, the capital of Phuoc Tuy province and home of Australian combat troops. This chapter will look at the work of the surgeons, nurses and other medical personnel, nearly 450 of them, who made up these teams.

By the early 1960s, the medical situation for the civilian population of South Vietnam, comprising approximately 16 million people, was dire. Of the country's 850 doctors, only 158 were available to care for civilians: the rest had been drafted into the army.[4] The country's 38 French-built provincial hospitals were run down, poorly staffed and lacked the capacity to carry out all but the most basic surgery. In desperation, the South Vietnamese government appealed to its allies to contribute medical and other civilian aid to help its people. In response, the US aid agency, USAID, began to greatly increase its medical aid contribution by constructing new surgical suites and improving existing facilities at hospitals throughout the country. USAID also made an international appeal for teams to carry out surgery at these hospitals. Surgical teams began arriving in South Vietnam from around 1963, from countries such as the United States, New Zealand, South Korea, the United Kingdom, the Philippines, China, France and Cuba. In addition, the large German hospital ship, the *Helgoland*, was moored in the Saigon River for several years.[5]

A request for Australian surgical assistance was relayed to the Department of External Affairs (DEA) in 1962. An exploratory mission by Melbourne neurologist Dr John Game recommended that Australia send one surgical team in the first instance. It took two years to organise this team, which came from the Royal Melbourne Hospital.

The surgical teams had three aims: (1) to provide a general surgical and medical service for the South Vietnamese; (2) to teach the Vietnamese medical staff, mainly by example; (3) to serve as evidence of Australia's support and concern for the people of South Vietnam.

Australia's surgical teams came under the administration of the DEA, rather than the Army, a point that was to become a source of frustration many years later. Team members were flown first class to Saigon via Singapore on diplomatic passports, and were given free food and accommodation in Vietnam, plus a small daily allowance. Nurses served between four months and a year, and surgeons between three and four months (although some surgeons did more). Many did multiple tours to Vietnam.

Reasons for joining a surgical team varied. For young single nurses it was a chance for adventure and the opportunity to see a new country. Some women, like Dorothy Angell, had already nursed overseas and wanted to continue the experience. Others wanted excitement, but also felt a need to help out civilians in war. Jenny Hunter was typical of some nurses in this regard; she had already nursed in Britain and thought that Vietnam would be an adventure, but she also felt she had a duty to go. As she commented, 'I was fit and well and a nurse', and that was sufficient reason to sign up.[6] For surgeons, doing a tour of duty in South Vietnam was seen as an opportunity to gain extra surgical skills, and to do some good in a war-torn country. Dr Peter Last was typical of some doctors who wanted to emulate their teachers, men who had worked as surgeons during the Second World War. He was too young to get involved in that war, and to have gone to Korea in the 1950s would have interrupted his medical studies. However, he always felt a sense of inadequacy that he had not had the experience of war, and going to Vietnam would give him that. It would give him a chance, he said, to look his veteran teachers in the eye.[7]

The manner in which the teams were assembled varied over time. Initially the major teaching hospitals from around the country were asked to provide teams. The first ones were small and included two surgeons, an anaesthetist, a physician, two theatre sisters, a ward sister and a radiographer. Later teams were larger and included up to five surgeons, more nurses, an administrator, a laboratory technician, a paediatrician and specialists such as plastic and orthopaedic surgeons, who rotated between teams. The largest teams were approximately sixteen men and women. A team leader was always appointed to manage the teams, and he was usually a senior surgeon. The team leader's role was vital. Not only was he responsible for the day-to-day running of the teams, but he also had to create team cohesion and maintain unity, often under very trying conditions. Occasionally, teams were led by uninspiring and divisive leaders who did more harm than good, but on the whole the team leaders did an excellent job. Their jobs became much easier with the addition of administrators, who took over the job of finding medical and food supplies, dealing with accommodation issues, and maintaining the teams' vehicles.

It is quite apparent that most surgical teams were poorly prepared for what they were to face. The DEA must take the blame for this situation. Briefings for team members by department officers were rudimentary and random and most received no briefing at all. On occasions some team members were flown to Canberra for a brief talk by DEA officials, while others were offered quick language courses in French, which they had been told would be sufficient for them to get by in Vietnam. Dorothy Angell was very blunt about the lack of preparation. As she commented in a filmed interview, 'the preparation we had was nothing. It was like a tour guide to sunny Vietnam. We had no idea what the living and working conditions would be like . . . And there was no discussion about what it would be like to be a woman in a war zone.'[8]

On most occasions, teams were given just a few weeks notice before they left. This time was taken up with vaccinations, buying suitable clothes, farewelling colleagues and family and, for those doctors who were in private practice, finding suitable locums to replace them. It was only due to the foresight of team members that so many arrived in Vietnam with enough supplies and equipment

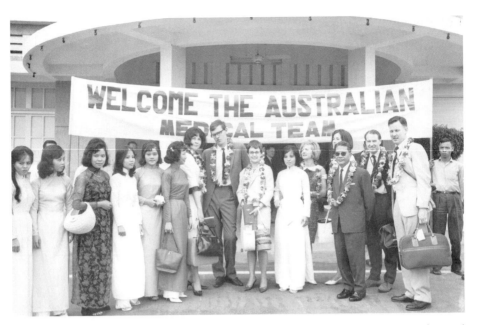

The first Australian civilian surgical team to South Vietnam being welcomed at Saigon's Tan Son Nhut airport on 4 October 1964. Over 450 Australian civilian medical and surgical staff volunteered to work in hospitals in South Vietnam during the war, where they provided medical treatment and instructed Vietnamese medical and paramedical personnel. (AWM P05373.003)

to allow them to start work. Getting adequate supplies of medical equipment and medicines was a constant problem for all teams. As time went on and later teams were advised of the problems, most carried substantial supplies to Vietnam with them, and then learned the valuable art of scrounging once their supplies ran out in the country. Although the Vietnamese were supposed to supply all foreign-aid teams from a depot in Saigon, the black market was rife and orders were either never filled or greatly delayed. If it were not for the vast stocks of medical supplies provided by American and Australian army hospitals, the Australian teams could not have operated.

The first surgical team, from Royal Melbourne Hospital, arrived in the Mekong Delta town and provincial capital Long Xuyen, in October 1964. The team received something of a heroes' welcome. A full media pack met the team at Saigon's Tan Son Nhut airport and smiling young women presented team members with garlands of fresh flowers. The Vietnamese Minister for Foreign Affairs and the Director General of Health greeted the team in front of a large welcome banner. The welcome continued in Long Xuyen, a pretty town in An Giang province on the banks of the Bassac River. Later teams were generally not welcomed as enthusiastically, although there is no doubt that the Vietnamese were very glad to have them.

An Giang province had a population of nearly half a million, but only seven doctors. The province and Long Xuyen itself was relatively free of Viet Cong activity, largely because of the prevalence of a religious sect called the Hoa Hao, a strongly anti-communist group which helped to keep the province safe. Nevertheless, Long Xuyen was close to the Cambodian border, where there was constant fighting.

Long Xuyen hospital was typical of provincial hospitals throughout South Vietnam. Made up of a series of pavilions, it was set in attractive tropical gardens and at first glance appeared quite pleasant. It was only when the Royal Melbourne team saw inside the buildings that they had misgivings. The 250-bed hospital regularly had nearly double that number of patients, crowded into dirty and very basic hospital wards. Almost no surgery was being carried out. Patient care was provided by relatives, who crowded into the halls and wards with their cooking and sleeping equipment. The Royal Melbourne team began work immediately, taking over the surgical suite and building up an outpatients clinic. This first team, like all those that followed, had to accept quickly that they were not in Long Xuyen to take over the running of the hospital. Each provincial hospital had a head doctor and a basic Vietnamese staff. The Australians usually took over the surgical suites, recovery wards, paediatrics ward and outpatients clinics. They had to adapt quickly to a very different way of doing things, trying to teach by example, and accepting that Western hospital practices were not always transferable to a Southeast Asian hospital. Flexibility was a key requirement.

The type of medical conditions the teams encountered varied, but included such cases as appendicitis and peritonitis, bowel obstructions and stomach ulcer perforations, often in very advanced stages, and diseases such as tuberculosis, typhoid, tetanus, malaria, haemorrhagic fever and dysentery. Because of the lack of available surgery, long-standing conditions such as very large goitres and advanced cancers, and cleft lips and palates were also regularly treated. In Long Xuyen, where life centred around the river, surgeons encountered the unusual problem of women being scalped when their hair became caught in outboard motor boat engines. All teams had to deal with a wide variety of war wounds, with bullet and grenade wounds being some of the most frequent. Some teams, like those in Bien Hoa, handled a far higher caseload of war-affected patients than others, but all teams experienced their share of civilians caught in the crossfire.

The teams also had to deal with the effects of Chinese or traditional medicine that the local population had come to rely on. Techniques such as cupping (where hot glasses were applied to the skin to draw the skin out into a protruding welt), the use of leeches to draw out infection and the application of cow dung poultices made many conditions worse, as did the long distances people had to travel to get to hospital.

The lack of a reliable source of blood was one of the most critical problems that all teams faced. Surgeons were often frustrated at losing patients because no stocks of matched blood were available, and all teams worked hard to boost supplies. Many team members, such as radiographer Noelle Laidlaw, donated their own blood when an emergency arose. Laidlaw helped save the life of a Vietnamese man brought to the Long Xuyen hospital with gunshot wounds to the abdomen. Without blood replacement, it was apparent the man would not survive for long, so she and some American servicemen donated enough blood to cover the surgery, thereby saving the man's life.[9] By donating her own blood, Laidlaw managed to convince the superstitious Vietnamese that it was a safe process, which enabled the team in Long Xuyen to begin developing a blood bank. In Bien Hoa teams relied more heavily on the huge US airbase nearby at Long Binh, with its enormous, well-stocked hospitals, for blood and other supplies. In Vung Tau and Ba Ria team members also donated their own blood, while American and Australian field hospitals also helped out.

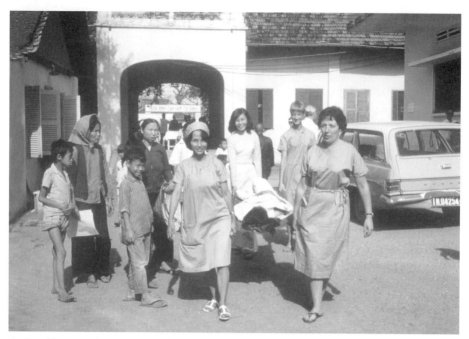

Assisted by two Vietnamese staff, Australian nurses, Sister Dorothy Angell (right rear) and Sister Pamela Matenson (right front), members of a surgical team from Alfred Hospital, Melbourne, transport a patient from the surgical suite to the recovery ward at Bien Hoa Hospital, South Vietnam, in early 1967. (AWM P03122.002)

For over 12 months rotating teams in Long Xuyen worked hard, establishing themselves in the hospital and gaining the confidence and respect of Vietnamese patients and staff. In early 1966 the Australian effort was expanded, when Melbourne's Alfred Hospital sent a team to Bien Hoa. This large and busy city, 25 kilometres north-east of Saigon, would be home to Australian surgical teams until their final withdrawal in December 1972. In an area surrounded by Viet Cong-controlled territory, the Bien Hoa hospital saw the largest caseloads of war-damaged patients, as well as many road accident victims. As the Alfred team was soon to discover, life in a Bien Hoa team was constantly hectic, and at times dangerous. Like all teams, the Alfred team was housed in an accommodation block not far from the hospital, with transport to the hospital either by jeep or on foot. The team was given little time to settle in at the hospital which was, like so many, dirty, crowded and lacking in even the most basic supplies.

The first team in Bien Hoa spent considerable time scrubbing the surgical suite just to make it usable. It encountered the same problems as the Long Xuyen teams, including intermittent power supplies, poor water supply, having to deal with the effects of Chinese medicine, treating advanced medical conditions with basic equipment and trying to communicate with Vietnamese staff, at times with no translators available. As a result of the Viet Cong presence in the area, Bien Hoa and the Long Binh airbase were frequently attacked. On several occasions surgeons at the hospital had their work interrupted when the Viet Cong exploded ammunition dumps or mortared the airbase. Hospital windows would be blown out and the power cut, but the surgeons would continue operating as best they could. At really busy times the Bien Hoa surgeons were conducting as many as 500 surgical procedures a month.

Danger came not only from the Viet Cong. On one occasion nurse Von Clinch, from the Alfred, was on duty in the evening when a truckload of South Vietnamese soldiers was brought in. They were normally treated at their own army hospitals so this was a bit unusual. Six stretcher cases were carried in and put on the floor; while they were being assessed, one of the men died. The soldiers who had brought them in were furious over this death; they pinned Clinch and a surgeon against a wall and held guns to their heads. Somehow the Australians managed to convey, in their limited Vietnamese, that if they were killed the rest of the Vietnamese soldiers would also die. And so they were allowed to continue working, albeit at gunpoint.[10]

At other times team members faced danger outside the hospital. The traffic in Bien Hoa was chaotic, and often just walking in the street was dangerous. Drunk and lonely American GIs on the loose also caused a problem for Australian nurses, although they were usually well protected by male team members. The teams also frequently had to brave the chaotic highway between Bien Hoa and Saigon, sometimes after curfew at night, and several were shot at. Their own team house came under fire on several occasions, especially during the 1968 Tet Offensive, and again during Tet in 1969.

The team that faced the greatest danger in Vietnam, however, was the one and only team sent to Ba Ria. That team, which arrived in late 1968, was a subsidiary of the first Vung Tau team, which arrived

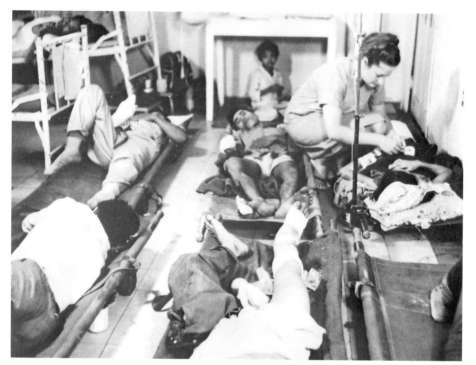

Sister Maureen McLeod, from an Australian civilian surgical team, checks the intravenous drip of a wounded Vietnamese patient lying on the floor of the recovery room at Bien Hoa Hospital, South Vietnam, 1966. In the crowded Vietnamese wards, it was common for numbers of patients to share beds and stretchers placed on the floor. (AWM P03122.001)

in the port town in November 1966. Vung Tau teams were sometimes seen by other teams, especially those in Bien Hoa, as having something of a holiday. Vung Tau, which was home to the Australian logistics support base and field hospital, was generally safe from Viet Cong attack. It also had some good beaches and other recreational facilities. Its hospital, however, was probably the most rundown of all those the Australians encountered. The first team in, from the Prince Henry and Prince of Wales hospitals, was led by eminent surgeon Professor Doug Tracy. The team spent its first two weeks scrubbing wards, despatching some very large rats, spraying insecticide and scrounging for basic supplies. Eventually, Tracy was able to begin surgery, but things did not start well when his very first patient, a young boy, died on the operating table from heat stroke. The non-functioning air conditioning meant that everyone in the operating theatre was so hot that the boy's condition, caused by an extreme reaction to anaesthetics, was not detected until it was too late. The team was so distraught that several members wanted to come home – but they didn't, and the Vung Tau teams slowly increased their caseload, in the process earning the trust of the local Vietnamese.[11] Surgeons such as Tom Hugh helped enormously, performing relatively simple but life-changing operations to repair cleft lips and palates, and removing large and ugly goitres. Patients who had lived with these conditions all their lives were extremely grateful to the teams.

The Ba Ria team was made up of personnel from Vung Tau and consisted of three doctors, three nurses and an anaesthetist. Ba Ria's hospital was only a small one but it was in the heart of heavily contested countryside and the team dealt with many victims of the war. Their greatest test came in 1969. In the early hours of 23 February team members were woken by American soldiers banging on their bedroom doors. They could hear the sounds of artillery and mortar fire outside, but this was not unusual. On this occasion, however, they were told that the rounds were incoming and the team was hurried into a purpose-built bunker in the grounds of their accommodation complex. They made it safely into the bunker but endured several hours of attack by Viet Cong, who threw grenades and directed automatic rifle fire at them. The team was protected by American and South Vietnamese forces, who put their lives on the line many times. The attack was over by dawn, and the team went back inside to shower and have a meal, before spending the day treating wounded civilians. They reported the details of the attack to the Australian ambassador in Saigon, and initially the Australian government agreed that they could stay on, despite the misgivings of some. Intelligence subsequently received by the Australian Army, however, showed that the Viet Cong had deliberately targeted the Australian team. It was considered too dangerous to have them remain so the hospital was taken over by a South Korean medical team, and the Australians either returned home or went to work in Vung Tau.[12]

Although the attack on the Ba Ria team was the only time an Australian team was deliberately targeted, other teams experienced threats. The Tet Offensive in January 1968 saw every major town and

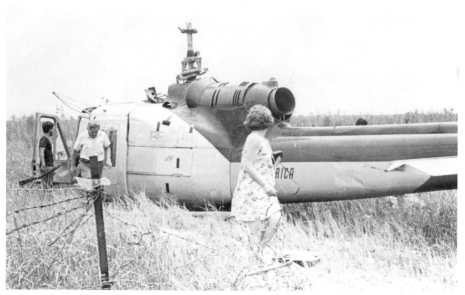

The work of the Australian surgical teams in Vietnam could still be hazardous, despite being civilians. Nurse Thelma Foxall and Australian consultant Ron Madden were on board this American Iroquois helicopter when it crash-landed after its rotor detached in early 1969. Neither was seriously wounded in the incident. (AWM P05519.001)

city in South Vietnam attacked by the Viet Cong and North Vietnamese forces. It was a busy and dangerous time. None of the teams' hospitals were directly attacked, but the caseload from civilians wounded in the offensive was enormous and continued for weeks. Several teams were given weapons by the US Army for protection, and the team in Long Xuyen took it in turns to stay on guard at night in the team's house. The team in Vung Tau worked itself to a standstill, and was eventually sent by the Vietnamese hospital staff to stay at the Australian logistics base for a rest. All teams were extremely relieved when the crisis passed and caseloads returned to something like normal.

Other dangers were often caused by the amount of air travel team members were required to do. Whether flying to visit one of the other teams, to Saigon to conduct business, or taking a joyride, team members became accustomed to flying in many different types of aircraft. Most of the flights were uneventful but there were incidents. Bien Hoa teams regularly travelled to the Ben San leprosarium, outside the city, to conduct surgery. On one occasion a team had finished its work and was heading back to Bien Hoa by Iroquois helicopter. On take-off a vital piece of the rotor failed and detached itself, causing the aircraft to crash heavily. Nurse Robyn Anderson was on board and she and a male surgeon grabbed the unconscious pilot and dragged him clear. The Viet Cong, alerted to the situation, appeared on the scene, causing team members to rush back to the leprosarium as fast as they could.[13]

For the final teams in Bien Hoa life became very dangerous. There were frequent rocket attacks near their accommodation, and operations at the hospital were often interrupted by nearby attacks. The Americans and other allies, including Australia, were withdrawing resources from South Vietnam, and so in a sense the teams were left on their own. By December 1972 the Australian government had decided to discontinue this form of aid to South Vietnam and the Australians handed a substantially improved Bien Hoa Hospital back to the Vietnamese on 28 December.

Naturally the stresses of working in such difficult conditions in a war zone took their toll. Team members socialised as hard as they worked, their relative youth enabling them to live a lifestyle that involved almost all work and play, and very little sleep. Female team members bore an extra load, often being required to entertain American army personnel in order to gain access to vital medical supplies, something many of them found arduous after a long day at work. Within the teams they held impromptu parties, wrote long letters home and formed lasting friendships. Many also formed close bonds with their Vietnamese colleagues, who were generous with their hospitality. Team members on longer tours were given rest and recreation breaks away, and many took the opportunity to travel to other Southeast Asian countries. Within South Vietnam, towns like Dalat, Nha Trang, Hue and Saigon were also popular destinations for a break. Team leaders tried to ensure that their team members had regular weekends off, with many visiting other teams; Vung Tau was a popular destination. As they had a diplomatic function, too, teams were regularly required to attend functions at the Australian embassy in Saigon, but apart from these occasions interest in and contact with teams by the Australian embassy appear to have been minimal.

When it came time to return home, most team members did so with mixed feelings. Those who had gone to Vietnam with high expectations of being able to make major and permanent improvements in the country's hospital system were inevitably disappointed. It is to their credit that many of the experienced surgeons and physicians who worked in Vietnam wanted to make a lasting difference and tried hard to do so. However, the DEA failed to emphasise that this was not the teams' role, and that temporary surgical and medical relief should be their primary goal. Those who had more limited and realistic expectations were generally more satisfied with their experience, and felt that they had made a difference to the lives of thousands of Vietnamese civilians. Nurse Jill Storch, who worked in two teams in Bien Hoa, summed up the feelings of many: 'in the face of their adversity I was really overwhelmed by the way they dealt with their life. I was very grateful for having experienced that regardless of what it did to me. I think it made me a better person.'[14]

In 1998, former team members had their service recognised by the Federal government when they were awarded the Australian Active Service Medal and the Vietnam Logistic and Support Medal. Two years later, Major General Justice Mohr was appointed to review service anomalies in respect of Southeast Asian service. The review included an investigation of team members' claims that they should be brought under the Veterans' Entitlements Act in order to be able to claim repatriation benefits. Many of them were suffering from the same illnesses and mental health issues as their military counterparts, without the benefit of having a military Gold Card.[15] Justice Mohr agreed with their claim, recommending that they be deemed as having performed qualifying service for repatriation benefits. In Federal Parliament, Democrat Senator Natasha Stott Despoja said:

> These civilian doctors and nurses assisted the Australian defence forces in wartime, and they incurred danger from hostile enemy forces during that time. They have a right to apply for repatriation entitlements under the Veterans' Entitlements Act.[16]

Labor Senators Chris Schacht and John Hogg, members of the Senate Foreign Affairs, Defence and Trade Legislation Committee, also recommended that team members 'be deemed as performing qualifying service for repatriation benefits'.

The Federal government disagreed, arguing that because the teams were in Vietnam under the auspices of the DEA (Department of Foreign Affairs from November 1970), rather than as part of the military, they would not be eligible for repatriation benefits.

Bitterly disappointed, team members led by Dorothy Angell tried again in 2002 to have their case recognised. In that instance, the Review of Veterans' Entitlements, chaired by the Hon. John Clarke, QC, overturned the recommendation by Justice Mohr in 2000. This left team members only one avenue to pursue compensation for their health claims, through the Federal Government agency Comcare. Several have pursued this course but have found it lengthy, complicated and ultimately unsatisfactory. Team members, through their organisation, Civilian Nurses – Australian Surgical Teams Vietnam 1964–1972, have continued to campaign for inclusion under the Veterans' Entitlements Act, in the hope that future Federal governments will look more favourably on their case.

10

The official history's Agent Orange account: the veterans' perspective

Graham Walker

In 1965 the United States Air Force (USAF) was being frustrated. It had mastery of the skies over South Vietnam and wanted to unleash its air power on the local units of National Liberation Front (NLF) and on the troops of the People's Army of Vietnam (PAVN). But those enemies skilfully used the thick canopy of the Vietnamese jungle to avoid attack from the air. For the USAF the solution was clear: remove the canopy by defoliating the jungles with Agent Orange. This herbicide was also used for the destruction of enemy crops and for clearing lines of sight around bases and along the sides of roads.

The term 'Agent Orange' popularly refers to a number of chemical mixtures used in Vietnam as defoliants. Strictly speaking, it was the name of the most widely used of those defoliants, a mixture of the chemical 2,4,D and the chemical 2,4,5-T with its impurity, dioxin. Other herbicides to which servicemen and women were potentially exposed were picloram, cacodylic acid, diquat, paraquat, bromocil, borate chlorate and creosote.

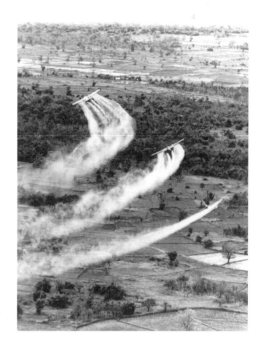

US Air Force aircraft spray defoliants over South Vietnam in 1969.
(Image courtesy of AAP)

Between 1965 and 1971, the USAF used low-flying aircraft to spray some 20 million US gallons (75.7 million litres) of these chemical agents over the Vietnamese countryside.[1]

The chemical deluge did not end there. In the tropical heat and humidity of South Vietnam, mosquitoes, spiders and scorpions thrived. To kill these and other pests in military bases, chemical insecticides such as DDT, malathion, lindane, chlordane and dieldrin were regularly sprayed from the air and ground, while soldiers engaged in night ambushes saturated themselves with insecticides from pressure packs. These insecticides are sometimes included under the banner of Agent Orange.

During the war, scientists in the United States began linking exposure to Agent Orange with cancer and birth defects. As a result, the herbicide spraying program was discontinued in 1971.

After the war, worried Australian veterans began to come together to ask about the chemicals to which they had been exposed and the possible consequences of that exposure. No satisfactory answers came from the Federal government and bureaucracy.

Disappointed by the official response, the veterans, headed by Phil Thompson and supported by Tim McCombe, Terry Loftus and others, began to make their own enquiries. Guided by scientific advice, they gathered evidence indicating that exposure might cause cancer, birth defects and toxic brain dysfunction. But they were aware that other credible studies had failed to confirm a causal link. This conflicting evidence produced doubt. But the veterans were confident that the Repatriation Commission would agree to provide treatment and compensation to sick veterans who had been exposed to Agent Orange, because repatriation law demanded that war veterans be given the benefit of such doubt.[2]

Such special consideration for war veterans was not new. With increasing numbers of servicemen returning from the First World War, the Australian Soldiers' Repatriation Bill was introduced into parliament by the Minister for Repatriation, Senator E.D. Millen, in 1917. Repatriation, the Minister said, was 'an earnest attempt to meet the nation's obligations to those who on its behalf have gone down into the Valley of the Shadow of Death'.[3] The bill included compensation arrangements and medical care specifically tailored for war-damaged veterans.

The Prime Minister at that time, Billy Hughes, had no doubts that this obligation was the result of an unwritten but binding contract between the Australian parliament and Australia's servicemen and women: '[W]e say to them "You go and fight, and when you come back we will look after your welfare". . . [W]e have entered into a bargain with the soldier, and we must keep it.'[4] Hughes made it clear that the servicemen and women had every right to expect that the government would honour its promises: 'The soldier will say to the Commonwealth Government. "You made us a promise. We look to you to carry it out."'[5]

By 1929 it had become clear that too great a burden was being placed on returned servicemen in seeking compensation for war-related disabilities. The remedy was the Australian Soldiers' Repatriation Act 1929, which relaxed evidentiary rules and put the onus on the Repatriation Commission to disprove a veteran's prima facie case.

In 1941 the Federal parliament again considered its responsibilities to the members of the armed forces returning from the front. A

Joint Parliamentary Committee examined the adequacy of existing repatriation arrangements 'in the light of the conditions caused by the 1939 war'[6] and under the pressure of some 'well publicised grievances'[7] generated by the existing legislation. The result was Australia's new repatriation contract with its fighting forces, as embodied in the Australian Soldiers' Repatriation Act 1943.

In framing the new Act, much thought was given again to how difficult it should be for sick and disabled veterans to have their illnesses and disabilities accepted as war-caused. The thought of sick war veterans having to continue to fight their way through court hearing after court hearing, with too heavy a burden of proof on them, was abhorrent both to the parliament and to the Australian people. So the new legislation included a more lenient test for whether a veteran's sickness could be linked with war service. In short, the new legislation gave veterans a generous 'benefit of the doubt'. In introducing the legislation, the Attorney-General explained:

> . . . if any question which is material to the case before any of these tribunals cannot be placed <u>beyond doubt</u>, the question must be determined in favour of the member of the forces . . . The whole purpose of this provision is to reverse completely the method of proof and to put the burden of proof upon the authorities to negative any connection between war service and the disability.[8]

During the long parliamentary debate on the 1943 bill, the Federal Opposition's only objection to this provision was that it might not be generous enough.[9]

While successive Federal parliaments supported these provisions, ambiguities in the wording of the Act led to disputes between the Repatriation Commission and the veteran community over interpretation of the 'benefit of the doubt' rule.

In 1977, however, parliament settled this issue in an amendment to the Act. In unambiguous wording that closely reflected the Attorney-General's 1943 explanation, the parliament reiterated its intention that the 'benefit of the doubt' rule should be interpreted generously.[10] Senator Peter Durack, the Minister for Veterans' Affairs responsible for the amendment, later told parliament: 'In redrafting the legislation, we gave the right of [reverse onus of] proof beyond reasonable doubt, which is now enshrined in the Act, to veterans.'[11]

It was in this longstanding tradition of what Billy Hughes had described as the 'bargain', the 'promise', that Vietnam veterans began applying for compensation for cancer on the grounds that it may have been caused by their exposure to Agent Orange. The veterans were acting as Hughes had predicted they would: 'The soldier will say to the Commonwealth Government: "You made us a promise. We look to you to carry it out."'[12]

The Repatriation Commission rejected the veterans' claims. The veterans believed this was because the Repatriation Commission had failed to concede the 'benefit of the doubt', as prescribed by law. This belief was reinforced by the large (and increasing) numbers of veterans whose compensation claims were initially rejected but who were subsequently successful at appeals tribunal hearings. In 1982–83, for example, 87 per cent of appeals to the Repatriation Review Tribunal were successful.[13] One of these successful appeals, which the campaigning veterans sponsored, was the Colin Simpson case. In 1982 the Repatriation Review Tribunal found that Simpson's fatal lymphoma was caused by his exposure to Agent Orange.

Frustrated at the Repatriation Commission's behaviour, and wanting all available evidence to be gathered, the veterans demanded an enquiry by a Royal Commission. After a change of government in 1983, the Evatt Royal Commission began its enquiry.[14]

An article in the April 1983 edition of the Vietnam Veterans' Association's journal *Debrief* canvassed the Evatt enquiry's possible outcomes. It said in part:

> It is possible that the Royal Commission could recognise that substantial conflicting evidence exists, therefore leaving the question in doubt. In this case the Department's policy of not accepting chemical exposure as the cause of certain

disabilities would be shown to be wrong because it is the Department's obligation to give veterans the benefit of any doubt. [15]

The Evatt enquiry's report was presented in 1985. It confirmed the suspicions of the campaigning veterans:

> It is a matter of public record that there has been a clear divergence of opinion and of result between the Repatriation Review Tribunal and the Repatriation Commission as to the proper interpretation and application of the standards of proof prescribed under the legislation.[16]

The enquiry was clear on who was guilty of error. It noted that the Repatriation Commission had 'for a number of years, refused to concede that benevolent judicial interpretations of the application of . . . [the law] were consistent with parliamentary intention'.[17] And, the report said, the Department was guilty of 'finding a method whereby the Repatriation Commission may restrict benefits which have flowed from a generous – though proper – interpretation of the legislation'.[18]

The Evatt enquiry went so far as to accuse the Repatriation Commission of training Determining Officers 'to find ways around Court statements of what the law was'[19] and of emphasising 'ways in which a claim could be "knocked-out"'.[20]

In May 1985, while the Evatt enquiry was still sitting, an amendment was made to repatriation law that made it more difficult for veterans to succeed in claiming compensation.[21] The amendment introduced a more onerous standard of proof, requiring veterans' evidence to pass a 'reasonable hypothesis' test before the 'benefit of the doubt' could be given. Within a year the success rate of veterans' claims had declined.[22]

It was in the light of this less generous legislation that the Evatt enquiry made its medical findings. It found no link at all between exposure to Agent Orange and birth defects or toxic brain dysfunction. However, in the body of the report, the Evatt enquiry, despite the new evidentiary hurdle in repatriation law, did find a link between exposure to Agent Orange and some cancers. Specifically, it found that a repatriation-determining authority might well attribute a Vietnam veteran's soft-tissue sarcoma or non-Hodgkin's lymphoma to his exposure to Agent Orange while on war service in Vietnam.[23] Had the 1985 amendment not been enacted, the list of cancers would most likely have been longer.

Confusingly for some, the 'Conclusions and Recommendations' section of the enquiry's report failed to mention the link with soft-tissue sarcoma and lymphoma. Indeed in its summing-up, the report proclaimed: 'There is no reliable evidence that the chemicals in Agent Orange cause cancer in humans.'[24] In general, it declared 'Agent Orange Not Guilty'.[25]

Clearly the 'Not Guilty' findings were made at a higher standard of proof than that demanded in repatriation legislation.[26] Those conclusions were, therefore, irrelevant to the veterans' case. Nevertheless, the Repatriation Commission focused only on the 'Not Guilty' conclusions and continued to reject veterans' cancer claims.

The greater propensity of the two appeals tribunals to obey the law had been noted both by the campaigning veterans and the Evatt enquiry. And so, disappointed with the Repatriation Commission's continuing intransigence, the veterans turned again to sponsoring appeals. Of course, the 1985 amendment made success more difficult to achieve, but assisted by the mountain of information compiled by the Evatt enquiry and supported by eminent medical scientists, the campaigning veterans sponsored successful case after successful case.

The first of these successful cases heard by the Administrative Appeals Tribunal was the Adrian Crisp case.[27] He was an infantry soldier in Vietnam who later died from malignant schwannoma (cancer of the nerve sheath). In 1990 the Tribunal found that Crisp's cancer had been caused by his exposure to toxic chemicals during his Vietnam tour of duty. In 1991 the Tribunal accepted veteran John Humffray's[28] death from astrocytoma (a cancerous tumour of the brain) as chemically caused. Later in 1991 the Tribunal found

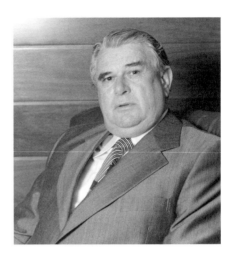

Royal Commissioner Justice Phillip Evatt who, from 1983 to 1985, oversaw the major investigation into the use and effects of chemical agents on Australian personnel in Vietnam.

(Image courtesy of Federal Court of Australia.)

that veteran Michael Shar's[29] pituitary adenoma (a cancerous tumour of the pituitary gland) had been caused by his exposure to herbicides. There were also the cases of Peter Edwards and Ken Kain, heard jointly.[30] In December 1992 the Tribunal found that both veterans' Hodgkin's lymphoma had been caused by their exposure to toxic chemicals while in Vietnam.

There were also a number of cases conceded by the Repatriation Commission before hearings at the Administrative Appeals Tribunal. Additionally, more than ten cases were won at the first level of appeal, the Veterans Review Board.[31] The Repatriation Commission, seemingly at war with the law, the appeals tribunals and the intentions of parliament, was continuing to resist stubbornly.

Meanwhile, an historian, Professor F.B. Smith, was chronicling the Agent Orange controversy for the official history of the Vietnam War. In early 1994 his account was published in the official history's third volume, *Medicine at War*.[32] Smith unreservedly supported the Evatt enquiry's 'Not Guilty' conclusions and vigorously castigated those who questioned them. His account, however, was silent on the events directly relevant to the veterans' case. There was no mention of the Evatt enquiry's finding that, given the 'benefit of the doubt' required by law, some cancers could be linked with veterans' exposure to Agent Orange. Missing too was any reference to the Evatt enquiry's rebuke to the Repatriation Commission for its systematic attempts to circumvent the 'benefit of the doubt' provision.

And what did Smith make of the appeals tribunal hearings that time and time again found veterans' cancers could be attributed to their exposure to Agent Orange, hearings that for some eight years had tested the evidence and found it convincing?[33] In this, Smith seems to have joined the Repatriation Commission in its war on the law, the appeals tribunals and the intentions of parliament because he mentions only two of these appeals tribunal hearings and then only to dismiss their importance, complaining that the veterans' success depended on them being given the benefit of the doubt.[34]

These omissions were startling. They showed that Smith had failed to identify the core of the controversy. The story that Smith missed can be summed up as follows. The Repatriation Commission repeatedly rejected veterans' claims that they may have been harmed by their exposure to Agent Orange. The veterans believed those claims were being rejected mainly because the Repatriation Commission failed to give the 'benefit of the doubt' as required by law. Their suspicions were confirmed by the Evatt enquiry, which reprimanded the Repatriation Commission for wilfully circumventing this law. While the Evatt enquiry was sitting, a legislative amendment was passed that made it more difficult for veterans' compensation claims to succeed. Despite this added difficulty, the Evatt enquiry found that, under repatriation law, soft-tissue sarcoma (with its very many varieties) and lymphoma could be linked with exposure to Agent Orange in Vietnam. Subsequently, the campaigning veterans, time and time again, sponsored cases at the appeals tribunals in which veterans' cancers were attributed to Agent Orange exposure.

Surely this meant that the veterans were vindicated in their 'David and Goliath' contest with the Repatriation Commission. But rather than acknowledge the veterans' success in that contest, Smith launched an attack on the veterans' leadership. Professor Smith had a belief about the 1980s. It was a time, he proclaimed, 'when … private greed became, for some, a public good'.[35] Without interviewing any of the campaign's national leaders, he lumped them into that category. In intemperate outbursts, he declared: 'A small minority of disgruntled Vietnam veterans seized on the issue both as an explanation of their discontent and a likely source of [undeserved] additional repatriation benefits.'[36] For Smith, '[t]he clash epitomizes many of the worst aspects of Australian behaviour in the 1980s.'[37]

But was this really true of the national leadership? Had they not already given the most selfless service possible: going to war on behalf of the Australian community?

Phil Thompson was the campaign's national leader. He was later awarded a Medal of the Order of Australia (OAM). He completed two tours of Vietnam with the 1st Battalion, Royal Australian Regiment (1RAR), during which he fought at the battle of Fire Support Base Coral and was later wounded by rocket-propelled grenade shrapnel. He was devastated when, after 14 years' service, he was discharged from the army at the rank of warrant officer with a hereditary cancer. He saw his leadership of the Vietnam veteran movement as a continuation of his service.

Tim McCombe was one of the national leadership team. He also was later awarded a Medal of the Order of Australia. He served with 2RAR in Vietnam, where he lost a leg after standing on a mine. McCombe has for many years served the veteran community as the National President of the Vietnam Veterans' Federation of Australia.

Terry Loftus was another member of the national leadership team. He served two tours in Vietnam with 1RAR, during which he was wounded in action and Mentioned in Despatches. He left the army as a warrant officer after 22 years' service. Since the early 1980s, Loftus has given continuous service to the veteran community. There were others among the national campaign leadership of the same ilk. So at the time of publication, Smith's story of the veterans' Agent Orange campaign was not only fatally flawed, it was also insulting.

Since then, the credibility of Smith's account has continued to crumble. In July 1993, the US National Academy of Sciences released a report (commissioned by the US Congress) on the association between Agent Orange exposure during Vietnam service and ill health.[38] The National Academy of Sciences had reviewed all existing publicly available evidence. It concluded, at a demandingly high standard of proof, that exposure to Agent Orange was associated with several kinds of cancer.[39] It effectively overturned the Evatt enquiry's conclusion that '[t]here is no reliable evidence that the chemicals in Agent Orange cause cancer in humans',[40] and thus cast doubt on the 'Not Guilty' conclusion.

Although the US National Academy of Sciences report was published some seven months before the publication of *Medicine at War*, there was no mention of it in Professor Smith's account. Perhaps seven months before publication had been too late in the publishing process to make changes to his manuscript. But even after the release of the US National Academy of Sciences report, Smith still did not publicly modify his position. And when interviewed for the March 1994 edition of the *Bulletin*, he failed to acknowledge the US report's findings.[41] This was another of his strange silences.

Following up on the 1993 publication of the US National Academy of Sciences report, the Australian government commissioned a review of it.[42] Published in 1994, the review concluded that, at a high standard of proof,[43] the following cancers were linked with exposure to Agent Orange: soft-tissue sarcoma (with its very many varieties); non-Hodgkin's lymphoma; Hodgkin's disease; multiple myeloma; leukemia; and respiratory cancers (lung, larynx, trachea). It also concluded there was strong evidence for a link with chloracne and porphyria cutanea tarda.

Subsequently, the Australian repatriation system accepted these cancers and diseases as 'war-caused' in Vietnam veterans who stayed a minimum period in-country, thus entitling them to medical treatment and compensation. As a result of further US and Australian reports, prostate cancer, type 2 diabetes (subject to a blood test) as well as acute and sub-acute transient peripheral neuropathy were added to the list.

And what of birth defects? Professor Smith strongly supported the Evatt enquiry finding, which had stated: 'The hypothesis that exposure of fathers to chemicals in Vietnam caused birth defects in children conceived in Australia is fanciful'.[44] However, the 1996 update of the US National Academy of Sciences report challenged this finding.[45] The report identified a link between exposure of veteran fathers to Agent Orange and their children suffering the birth defect spina bifida. While the report did not put the strength of evidence in the highest category, the evidence was sufficiently compelling for the US government to accept responsibility and generously compensate the affected children.[46] In other words, the hypothesis of a link between the fathers' exposure to Agent Orange and birth defects in their children is far from 'fanciful'.

Indeed, the US report's 2008 update strengthened the possibility of a link with birth defects. It stated that the developing understanding of the transgenerational effects of Agent Orange was making the link between fathers' exposure and their children's ill-health more plausible, and recommended increasing the level of epidemiological research.[47]

In his account, Smith quoted the Australian Commonwealth Institute of Health birth defects study of 1983.[48] That study found that there was 'no evidence that army service in Vietnam increases the risk of fathering children with abnormalities diagnosed at birth'.[49] In 1997, however, an Australian government study found an increase in the incidence of spina bifida manifesta, cleft lip, cleft palate, adrenal gland cancer and acute myeloid leukemia in the children of Vietnam veterans.[50] The study was not specifically designed to find a link between the children's ill health and Agent Orange but it did establish a firm relationship with 'service in Vietnam'. The Australian government instituted a program of help for the victims.

The Agent Orange controversy was a chaotic episode. Given the horror of a situation in which veterans saw possible connections between their war service and a range of postwar cancers and birth defects, it was understandable that emotion sometimes overwhelmed rationality. In fact, as war-caused psychological stress sometimes amplified the concerns of veterans, their claims could become exaggerated and even hysterical. The pronouncements of some over-enthusiastic lawyers and fringe medicos did not help either. Additionally, the media fed an intense public interest with sensational and sometimes inaccurate reports. There were also problems with the evidence presented to the Evatt Royal Commission. In some cases, the scientific opinions on which the veterans had relied were cut to pieces. In one case, a witness was even found to have exaggerated his qualifications. The evidence given by some Vietnam veterans was also found to be flawed and unconvincing.

Smith spends a large proportion of his account indignantly detailing these inaccuracies, exaggerations, ratbaggery and disappointments. Perhaps he was attracted to this detail because he felt it demonstrated his view that the 1980s was a time in Australian society when, as he put it, 'private greed became, for some, a public good'. But Smith's focus on these details seems to have blinded him to what was important. After all, the Evatt enquiry, the decision-makers and appeals tribunals of the repatriation system, and the courts were well equipped to sort out the wheat from the chaff. What was important were the findings of these enquiries and tribunals as they affected the veterans' case. Yet the most important of these findings, Smith entirely omits from his account. He gives us a comprehensive description of the static but misses completely the message.

It was not only these irrelevant details which distracted Professor Smith. He spends another large proportion of his account attempting to discredit those who disagreed with the Evatt enquiry's 'Not Guilty' verdict. In doing so, however, he failed to acknowledge that the 'Not Guilty' verdict was reached using a standard of proof irrelevant to the veterans' case. Smith's zeal in this pursuit may have been the reason he missed entirely the central finding of the Evatt enquiry that, under repatriation law, there was indeed a link between exposure to Agent Orange and certain cancers suffered by veterans.

Perhaps Smith also became blind to the core story because of his personal antipathy to the 'benefit of the doubt' law. He makes his disapproval of it clear. The chapter titled 'The Cancer Allegations' culminates in his criticism of the law's generosity to veterans in Administrative Appeals Tribunals decisions. Indeed, the chapter seems to have that criticism as its purpose. It is a puzzling attitude. The Evatt enquiry, which Smith believed was 'the pre-eminently thorough, authoritative survey of the Agent Orange episode',[51] found that the application of the law by the appeals tribunals was both consistent with 'parliamentary intention' and, whilst generous, was properly so. Moreover, a whole system of appeals tribunals and courts existed to expertly interpret and apply the law. Smith seems to have missed the point that it was within a long-established institutional, legal and philosophical context that the veterans were prosecuting their case, and not in some open scientific forum. His personal disapproval of veterans being treated generously is disappointing but irrelevant.

These themes, pursued by Smith, were red herrings that led him further and further away from the core issues. They may provide interesting polemics for some other forum, but they do not belong in a historical account of the veterans' encounter with Agent Orange. What should have guided Smith in this official history was the sentiment expressed in 1917 by Senator Millen and Prime Minister Hughes, and endorsed by every subsequent Australian parliament: '[W]e have entered into a bargain with the soldier, and we must keep it.'[52]

The official history's account of Agent Orange controversy betrays this sentiment. It was fatally flawed when it was written, and has since been further discredited and superseded. Sadly, it remains the official version of these events. It must be rewritten.

Australia's Agent Orange story: a historian's perspective[1]

Peter Edwards

This is a tale of competing narratives (to use one of today's buzz-words). As Graham Walker's chapter has indicated, the narrative of Australia's Vietnam veterans' exposure to Agent Orange is along the following lines. A group of Vietnam veterans in Australia, backed by some scientists, formed the Vietnam Veterans' Association of Australia (VVAA), who took up the cause that had originated with some of their fellow veterans in the United States. They asserted that exposure to dioxins in herbicides used as defoliants in Vietnam, often known collectively as Agent Orange, had led to a large number of physical and psychological ailments, including several cancers and even birth defects in their children. Despite several rebuffs, the VVAA succeeded in having a Royal Commission appointed by the Hawke government. To the great disappointment of VVAA members, however, the Royal Commissioner (Justice Phillip Evatt) rejected the VVAA case and accepted the opposing case presented by a major chemical company. In 1994 the section of the official Vietnam War history on Agent Orange, written by Professor F.B. Smith, was published, with high praise for the Royal Commission's conduct and report.[2]

At about the same time, however, a new report by the US National Academy of Sciences (NAS) reassessed the evidence and established a link between herbicides and certain cancers. This report, the narrative continues, 'overturned' all the previous rejections, including that of the Australian Royal Commission. A new Australian scientific report established that the American findings were applicable to Australian veterans. Thus the VVAA approach was completely vindicated, and this group of Australian veterans has asserted ever since that the Smith essay in the official history should be withdrawn and rewritten in a manner favourable to their narrative.[3]

This chapter suggests that there is another way to tell the story, with a particular focus on the reports in the early 1990s that supposedly 'overturned' the previous rejections. It addresses three questions. Why was the VVAA approach rejected for so long, before the NAS report of 1994? Did that report really 'overturn' all the previous rejections? And what have we learnt in the 15 years since then about the Agent Orange issue? What follows is another perspective, an alternative narrative.

The Agent Orange controversy originated with complaints by some American scientists while the war was still on, and was re-inforced by the allegations of the Vietnamese communist authorities that herbicides had caused widespread birth defects and other ailments. A group of Swedish scientists from the late 1970s linked soft-tissue cancers among forestry workers to exposure to the suspect chemicals. The controversy was further fuelled by reports that appeared after an explosive release of dioxins from a chemical factory in Seveso, near Milan. The argument was taken up by some Vietnam veterans in the United States and then in Australia, where the Vietnam Veterans' Action Association, soon renamed the Vietnam Veterans' Association of Australia, was founded in 1979–80, specifically to press the Agent Orange case. In Australia, as in the United States, the cause was supported by some scientists, activists, writers, journalists and politicians.

Although the veterans who took up this cause, especially in Australia, varied widely in their attitudes towards both the war and the anti-war protesters, much of the support for the Agent Orange campaign came from journalists, activists and politicians who had long been opposed to the war. The campaign resonated particularly with those who were keen to establish that Vietnam was not just another war, but an especially 'dirty' one. During the war its opponents had particularly criticised the use by US forces of napalm, a highly flammable petroleum jelly which inflicted horrific burns on its victims. A photograph of a naked Vietnamese girl, screaming from her napalm burns, became one of the emblematic images of the Vietnam War. To many in the anti-war movement, the use of napalm against Vietnamese villages made US chemical companies, such as Dow and Monsanto, major accomplices of the US government and its allies in what the protesters regarded as an immoral war. Since some of the same companies had been involved in the manufacture of the herbicides used in Vietnam, anti-war activists and disaffected veterans, especially in the United States, found common ground in their willingness to target the huge chemical companies. In this narrative, not only did the American forces use vicious forms of technological power with horrendous effects on the Vietnamese people and their environment, but they also destroyed the health of many of their own servicemen in this especially dirty and immoral war.

In the climate of the late 1970s and early 1980s, when anything associated with the American effort in Vietnam was seen as discredited, this appeared to be a powerful campaign with an influential coalition of supporters. But, if we seek to set aside the emotions associated with this highly emotive subject and analyse it cold-bloodedly as a political strategy, it can be seen to have several major flaws.

First, and most importantly, the approach depended on proving scientifically the case for linking exposure to the relevant herbicides to a wide range of physical and psychic ailments. It was one thing to assert that there was good reason to suspect that Agent Orange might well be linked to some of the veterans' postwar ailments, but quite another to prove, to scientifically reputable standards, a causal relationship between the dioxins in the herbicides and the extensive range of diseases of mind and body to which the veterans, and their offspring, were prone. There were at least four major obstacles in the way of establishing such causal relationships. First, too few persons had been definitely exposed to establish causality; second, too little time had passed for some long-latency diseases to have become evident; third, it was extremely difficult to single out the effects of the suspect chemicals from those of other potential causes of ill-health; and fourth, and most importantly in this context, it was too difficult to quantify exposure, so that scientists could establish a 'dose-response' or a 'dose-time-response' relationship between herbicide exposure and Vietnam veterans.

In addition to these scientific hurdles, the Agent Orange claim faced other problems. It put the discussion of compensation for war service-related ailments into an arena which posed greater difficulties. At a time when Australia was adopting American terms such as 'veteran' and 'Department of Veterans' Affairs' in place of 'returned servicemen' and 'Repatriation Department', the campaign adopted an American rather than an Australian approach to repatriation benefits. The Australian tradition, since the First World War, has been of the 'returned men' saying to government (in the broadest sense): 'We answered the call; you sent us in harm's way; we have suffered from our war service; you should give us fair treatment.' The official response has traditionally been generous, establishing a system of war pensions and benefits, and placing the onus of proof on the government to prove that a claim for compensation was *not* valid. Governments know that the electorate has always supported a generous attitude towards repatriation benefits. Moreover, what we might call the political-military establishment – defence planners, both uniformed and civilian, and politicians with a long-term view – know that recruitment and popular support for military commitments are closely associated with a strong tradition of postwar recognition and support for veterans and their dependants.

Within this political environment, the Australian approach towards generic complaints has been to compare rates of ailments between veterans and control groups of non-veterans. Where the veterans suffered significantly higher rates of an ailment, there was a prima facie case that the ailment was service-related, irrespective of the particular cause.

The Agent Orange lobby's approach was quite different. It took the American approach of identifying not only a wide range of ailments, but also the alleged cause and thus a specific body from which to seek compensation – in this case, the large chemical companies such as Dow and Monsanto. They must have been attractive targets. Their reputation was already tainted by their association with napalm and they were financially strong: there is no point in seeking recompense from the bankrupt. But this approach mobilised a powerful enemy. While the chemical companies had deep pockets, they also had long experience in using their resources to deploy the best legal and scientific expertise, not to mention political influence, in defence of their shareholders' interests. Instead of placing their claims in the hands of the political-military establishment, which has a strong interest in being seen to be fair to the point of generosity, the Agent Orange lobby was provoking a political battle with tough antagonists with the motivation, the resources and the experience to fight a powerful counter-campaign.

Major ex-service organisations, most importantly the Returned Services League (RSL), then led by the highly astute Sir William Keys, were well aware of the faults and the dangers in the Agent Orange lobby's approach. They could see that the Agent Orange campaign was likely to prove a distraction and distortion of the process governing compensation for those who served in Vietnam, tending to narrow rather than to broaden the grounds on which veterans might receive compensation. More generally, the Agent Orange campaign emphasised differences between Vietnam and other wars. Only Vietnam, it asserted, had the Agent Orange factor, only Vietnam was an especially dirty war. But many veterans, whether linked to the RSL, or the great majority who joined no organisation, wanted to be treated as similarly as possible to those who had served in the two world wars and other conflicts. Some said explicitly that they wanted to be included in the Anzac tradition, not to be seen as a group apart. There were many who resented the contribution that the Agent Orange campaign made towards making 'Vietnam veteran' a shorthand expression for someone who was seriously troubled in mind and body, instead of someone who was getting on with his postwar life, often in a responsible career.

Therefore, when considered in its scientific, legal, social and political contexts, the Agent Orange campaign can be seen as flawed. The ailing veterans needed a campaign based on reconciliation, unification and inclusion. Such a campaign would have said, in effect: 'Whatever you think of the rights and wrongs of the war, we deserve to be treated with the same respect and compassion as those who returned from service in Australia's previous wars. We should be compensated for service-related ailments, whatever their cause – and don't overlook herbicides among all the other possible causes.' Instead a campaign that placed overwhelming emphasis on the herbicides was confrontational, divisive and exclusive. It split veterans' organisations and the wider community of veterans; it divided politicians and political parties; and it divided scientists, as many of the most respected and authoritative bodies kept reasserting how hard it was to prove, or for that matter to disprove, the Agent Orange claims. It seemed that there was always just enough evidence to keep the issue alive, but not enough to establish the case to scientifically acceptable standards.

Given all these hurdles, scientific and other, it was not surprising that inquiry after inquiry, report after report, rejected the campaign's claims. As F.B. Smith pointed out in his essay, it was often the case that people came to these inquiries with an initial sympathy for the claimants, but became convinced by the evidence that the campaigners could not sustain their claim that herbicides were the predominant cause of a wide range of physical and mental ailments. Nevertheless, the VVAA and sympathetic Labor members ensured that a commitment was made before the 1983 election that a Labor government would establish a Royal Commission. The Hawke Labor government implemented this promise within weeks of its election, appointing Mr Justice Phillip Evatt as Royal Commissioner with

John Coombs QC as the counsel assisting. Both were well qualified for their roles but the appointments – a relative of H.V. 'Doc' Evatt, Clive Evatt and Elizabeth Evatt and a son of H.C. 'Nugget' Coombs – indicated that the new Minister for Veterans' Affairs, Senator Arthur Gietzelt, expected a report that would be authoritative, but as sympathetic as reasonably possible to the VVAA claims.

At the same time, the government and its advisers also included politicians, officials and scientists who were sceptical of many of the claims made by the VVAA and its sympathisers, and who were aware of an obligation to protect the public purse from open-ended compensation claims. One of the most significant of these was Senator Peter Walsh, the Minister for Finance from 1984 to 1990. Although his entry into politics had been prompted by his deep opposition to the Vietnam War, he was an exceptionally tough-minded defender of the public purse. He doubted whether a Department of Veterans' Affairs was even necessary and was often scathingly critical of expenditure proposals emanating from the party's left wing, especially Senator Gietzelt, whom he would later describe in his memoirs as 'one of the silliest people in Caucus'.[4]

Much of Smith's essay in the official history is based on a careful reading of the transcripts and reports of the Royal Commission. The report included nine volumes and 2760 pages, with over 360,000 words of text and 120,000 words in references. Smith praised the report as 'the pre-eminently thorough, authoritative survey of the Agent Orange episode'.[5] Much the same could be said of his own account of the Royal Commission's work. He hinted that, despite whatever inclinations they might have initially held to favour the VVAA claims, Evatt and Coombs, like others before them, may well have been converted by the evidence to the conclusion that Agent Orange was 'not guilty' of causing the diseases to which it had been linked (although at one point had suggested that there might be a case for a link with soft-tissue sarcomas). Smith even defended Evatt for phrasing his major conclusions in a populist style and for making extensive, and unacknowledged, use of the Monsanto submission in his report, two aspects which aroused considerable controversy. Unlike many other observers, Smith noted that, amid these controversies, Senator Gietzelt quietly rejected Evatt's recommendations that pensions should be paid to veterans suffering from alcoholism or from diseases caused by smoking.

Evatt's findings were clearly not what Senator Gietzelt had expected when he instituted the Royal Commission. Somewhat contradictorily, he said that he 'accepted' the Commission's argument, but that the government did not 'endorse' the findings. Making it quite clear that his problem was political rather than scientific or legal, Gietzelt took the unusual measure of referring the report to R.D. Hogg, a senior political adviser to the Prime Minister and long-standing Labor Party official. Hogg, while criticising Evatt for his unacknowledged use of the Monsanto submission, reported that the Royal Commission's findings were unchallengeable and should be accepted. Smith also recorded the quiet announcement in 1990 by Gietzelt's successor as Minister for Veterans' Affairs, Ben Humphreys, that the government accepted the Royal Commission's findings and 'equally unobtrusively rejected Hogg's recommendation supporting the Commissioner's proposal that repatriation benefits should cover circulatory disease, alcoholism and mental disorders'.[6]

There the matter rested in the early 1990s, when Smith was researching and writing his essay. Its publication in early 1994 provoked some media controversy. An article in *The Bulletin* described the 'bitter feud' that erupted. Smith's critics pointed to some recent reports that were more sympathetic to a possible link between exposure to herbicides and a small group of cancers. Smith did not resile from his perspective, drawing attention to the fact that the RSL had not entered the Royal Commission, warning the VVAA that its approach would serve only to narrow the grounds on which compensation would be granted to war veterans.[7] The last word in the *Bulletin* article was given to Professor John Mathews, who had been a scientific adviser to the Commission. He indicated that his only regret over Evatt's findings were that they were too uncompromising. Mathews stated that the evidence that Agent Orange caused cancer was still not strong enough to be sure, nor strong enough to exclude the possibility. His 'general conclusion [was] that most of the problems that worried the veterans after the Vietnam War weren't due to Agent Orange; they were just due to it being a bloody awful war'.[8]

Around this time the VVAA and its supporters pointed to various overseas reports, which were coming closer to concluding that exposure to herbicides might be linked to some forms of cancer. One particular report in the United States attracted huge attention. *Veterans and Agent Orange: Health Effects of Herbicides used in Vietnam* was commissioned from the Institute of Medicine within the NAS.[9] Worldwide attention was given to one of its conclusions, which linked exposure to herbicides to three forms of cancer and two skin diseases. The VVAA and scientists sympathetic to its cause asked why this report, which they asserted 'overturned' the Evatt Royal Commission report, had not been included in Smith's essay, which they alleged should be withdrawn and rewritten.

The answer to the question of the omission of this report, and its sequels, was a simple matter of timing. *Medicine at War*, a substantial book of 505 pages with extensive references and 21 statistical tables, took more than a year to pass through the publication process. It went to the publisher in late 1992 and emerged in March 1994. The NAS report was simply not available to Smith at the time he was writing.

The assertion that the NAS report 'overturned' the findings of the Evatt report (and all other reports which had been similarly sceptical of the link between herbicides and diseases among veterans) requires a more complex response. There are several important points about the NAS report that have generally been overlooked amid the extensive publicity given to one of its conclusions.

The NAS scientists were not asked to give advice on policies regarding compensation to Vietnam veterans, but there were numerous signs within their report that they were acutely conscious of the political, and the policy, context within which they were operating. They stated that the report had been initiated largely in response to continuing pressure by members of the US Congress, who were in turn responding to pressure from their constituents. The NAS scientists were also well aware of two important policy decisions that had already been made.

First, if scientists determined that the evidence supporting an association between a disease and exposure to a substance was equal to or greater than the evidence to the contrary, the Secretary of Veterans' Affairs would determine in favour of such a link being established. Second, if a veteran presented with one of the designated diseases, it would simply be presumed that the ailment was service-related.

In that context, the scientists were not asked to undertake a new research project themselves, but rather to carry out a review of the extensive literature in scientific journals on the possible association between herbicides and diseases, including cancer, birth defects and other ailments. The terms of reference were carefully framed. Their mandate was to determine: (1) whether there was a statistical association between the suspect diseases and herbicide use; (2) whether there was 'a plausible biologic mechanism' or other evidence of a causal relationship between herbicide exposure and a disease; and (3) the increased risk of disease among individuals exposed to herbicides in Vietnam.

After an extremely comprehensive inquiry, the committee issued a report of more than 800 pages. It divided diseases into four categories: (1) those with 'sufficient evidence' of an association between the diseases and herbicide use; (2) those with 'limited/suggestive evidence' of an association; (3) those where there was 'inadequate/insufficient evidence' to determine the existence of an association; and (4) those where there was 'limited/suggestive' evidence of no association. Into the first category were placed five diseases – three cancers (soft-tissue sarcoma, non-Hodgkin's lymphoma and Hodgkin's disease) and two skin diseases (chloracne and porphyria cutanea tarda). Three other cancers – respiratory cancers (lung, larynx and trachea), prostate cancer and multiple myeloma – were placed in the 'limited/suggestive category'. Amid all the publicity given to these conclusions, little attention was given to the long lists of diseases which were placed in the third and fourth categories.

The four categories were virtually the same as those used by authorities on cancer when assessing the carcinogenicity of specified substances. Their use therefore gave the impression that the NAS report was making conclusions about causality, when it was actually assessing the statistical evidence, together with evidence of a 'plausible biologic mechanism' – that is to say, important components in any assessment of causality, but not sufficient of themselves to pronounce on causality with the degree of certainty that scientists would wish.

The publicity given to the NAS report – indeed, its very title – led many to assume that this conclusion referred specifically to the link between the diseases listed and exposure to herbicides of servicemen in Vietnam. But on that term of reference, the NAS scientists said quite explicitly that they were unable to quantify the degree of risk to which the servicemen in Vietnam had been exposed. Despite numerous studies and reports, there was simply not enough reliable, quantitative evidence to draw any conclusions about the 'dose-time-response' relationship that might be applicable to Vietnam veterans. The NAS report stated that their statistical assessments were based on the scientific studies referring to Swedish forestry workers, North American agricultural workers, the residents of Seveso at the time of the explosion there, and others who had probably been exposed to far more of the herbicides in quantity and/or time than were most servicemen in Vietnam.

I suggest that what is actually happening here can fairly be characterised in the following way. Under pressure from Congress, the authorities in the United States framed the inquiry, and the policy settings within which it operated, in such a way as to maximise the opportunity for the scientists, without breaching their professional integrity, to give a degree of support to the claims made by the Agent Orange lobby, and thus to open the way to some compensation. The scientists, in a large, comprehensive and carefully worded report, gave what was in truth a limited and highly qualified response. They pointed to statistical and other evidence supporting a link between exposure to herbicides and a small number of the many diseases considered, but they stated explicitly that this was based on evidence concerning groups who had probably had far greater exposure to herbicides than most Vietnam veterans. Nevertheless, this was sufficient to allow the Agent Orange lobby to claim some success for their long campaign and for the authorities to open the door to some compensation to veterans. That compensation depended on the quiet acceptance of two huge assumptions, for which the policy settings had already been put in place: first, that what was true of groups exposed to large amounts of the herbicides was applicable to Vietnam servicemen; and, second, that if a Vietnam veteran presented with one of the specified diseases, he could claim that his ailment was service-related.

This is something rather different from the narrative of the dramatic overturning of all the previous rebuffs to the Agent Orange campaign. If one looks at the text, the subtext and the context, it is reasonable to draw the conclusion that the authorities were going to considerable lengths to create an escape route for the Agent Orange lobby from the obstacles posed by the path they had chosen. By carefully framing the terms of reference of the NAS inquiry, by putting the policy implications in the context of congressional sympathy for ailing veterans, by referring to the policies that gave veterans the benefit of any doubt, and by 'assuming' their way around two of the biggest obstacles to the finding that the Agent Orange campaigners wanted, the scientists and the officials created an opening towards some compensation for a limited number of Vietnam veterans.

When the NAS report appeared in 1994, the Labor government in Australia was still in office, although looking increasingly unlikely to survive the election due in early 1996. The then Minister for Veterans' Affairs, Con Sciacca, reacted quickly. He commissioned two scientists, Professors Robert MacLennan and Peter Smith, to report with the following terms of reference: (1) to examine the NAS report and comment on its 'scientific merit'; (2) to comment on the applicability of the report's findings to Australian veterans, especially of the diseases listed as 'limited/suggestive' of an association between exposure to herbicides and the disease and, if necessary, to assist in the preparation of Statements of Principles to address these diseases; and (3) to comment on the relevance of the report's recommendations to Australian veterans.

MacLennan and Smith also acted speedily, producing their report in September 1994.[10] Although it carried the same title as that of the NAS, it was far more modest in scope. Covering just 18 pages, it addressed its terms of reference succinctly. As to scientific merit, MacLennan and Smith concluded that the NAS report was 'a high quality review [of the scientific literature] by competent and respected scientists'; but they spent almost as much time on the references in the NAS report to the political and policy-making context as on the science. MacLennan and Smith also noted that the four categories were similar to those used to assess evidence of carcinogenicity, but used in the NAS report to assess statistical association, not causality.

The Australian scientists addressed the huge difficulties in gaining reliable evidence on the exposure of individual veterans to herbicides in Vietnam. As they explained, previous Australian reports, including one of which MacLennan himself had been a co-author, had attributed any difference in disease outcomes between veterans and control groups to Vietnam service, rather than linking it to one specific cause such as herbicide exposure. They drew attention to the NAS report's quite different approach, extrapolating the results of studies of highly exposed groups in other countries (such as the population of Seveso or the Swedish forestry workers) to the Vietnam veterans, whose degree of exposure was not quantifiable. MacLennan and Smith observed that this was 'giving the veterans the benefit of any doubt' and was apparently 'a response to the concerns of veterans'. They also noted, at some length, the NAS report's references to the two important American policies: first, that, if the credible medical and scientific evidence for an association between herbicides and disease in humans was equal to the credible evidence against the association, the Secretary of Veterans' Affairs would find in favour; and, secondly, that compensation policy would be based on a presumption that the association was based on war service. Here again, they observed, the veterans were being given the benefit of any doubt.

Having thus quite explicitly drawn attention to the political and policy context of the NAS report, and the differences between the American and previous Australian approaches to such issues, MacLennan and Smith proceeded to address the specific findings. They quickly endorsed the inclusion of the five diseases in the 'sufficient evidence' category. As required by their terms of reference, they devoted particular attention to the 'limited/suggestive' category. MacLennan and Smith contended that this category was unsatisfactory, not for scientific but for policy-making reasons, and deleted it. Two of the three cancers placed there by the NAS report, respiratory cancers and multiple myeloma, they moved up into the first category, 'sufficient evidence', while they moved prostate cancer down into the 'inadequate/insufficient evidence' category. Moreover, they moved leukaemia, which the NAS report had placed in the third or 'inadequate/insufficient evidence' category, to the top level of 'sufficient evidence'. They argued that the number of cases of leukaemia among non-smoking veterans would be small, and that they should be given 'the benefit of the doubt'.

Thus MacLennan and Smith had not only endorsed the conclusions of the NAS report but had extended the list of diseases in the 'sufficient evidence' category from five to eight: six forms of cancer and two skin diseases. The clear implication of their report was that, if the Australian government wished to give the veterans 'the benefit of the doubt' (a phrase that recurred frequently in their report), then not only would they have to endorse the generosity of the American approach, they would even have to extend it.

The speed and vigour of Minister Sciacca's response indicated that MacLennan and Smith had delivered precisely the sort of report for which he had hoped. In a media release, Sciacca stated that, while the NAS report had only concluded that 'there *could* be a link between some forms of cancer and herbicides, the Government has accepted the Australian doctors' recommendation that war veterans be given the benefit of the doubt'.[11] This, according to Sciacca, was in keeping with 'the generous nature of Australia's Repatriation system – recognised as one of the best, if not *the best* in the world'. Compensation claims from veterans and their widows for these cancers (Sciacca's statement inaccurately referred to the two skin diseases as cancers) would be 'fast-tracked', without waiting for the development of the usual 'Statements of Principles'. The enthusiasm of the minister for a solution to the government's longstanding political problem was almost palpable.

Not everyone in the political and scientific worlds shared

Sciacca's enthusiasm. His most caustic critic was Peter Walsh, the former Minister for Finance, who by this time had left Parliament and was writing acerbic columns for the *Australian Financial Review*. Walsh scathingly denounced the announcement, saying that Sciacca had secured an 'under-the-line' decision from Cabinet which required neither a Cabinet submission nor co-ordination comments from other departments and gave no opportunity for discussion. The number of such decisions was, in Walsh's view, 'an index of Cabinet decadence'. Walsh said that reports of the decision 'amounted to a media-inspired scientific fraud'. The extent of this fraud had been revealed by a Channel 9 *Sunday* program, which the print media had failed to report. In this, according to Walsh, MacLennan had said that there was no scientific evidence linking Agent Orange to cancer in Vietnam veterans, but 'they should administratively be regarded as service related'. In Walsh's view, MacLennan had thus 'jumped the fence from the scientific paddock ... into the political paddock'.

Walsh further reported that the *Sunday* program had quoted two other leading scientists in the field as stating that a few industrial workers might have experienced the high dosages of Agent Orange that could cause a small increase in cancers, 'there was neither scientific evidence nor rational reason to believe Vietnam veterans would be affected'. Walsh concluded:

> After parading his contempt for evidence and scientific method he [Sciacca] said: 'I'm going to give some peace of mind to those Vietnam veterans.' He is, in fact, feeding paranoia.[12]

Walsh's criticisms were unduly harsh on the scientists, who by their terms of reference and the general context had been invited, almost required, to 'jump into the political paddock'. In Australia, as in the United States, the political-bureaucratic sphere and the scientific sphere were collaborating to create an escape route for the Agent Orange campaign. The political context had simply been more obvious in the 18 pages of the MacLennan-Smith report than in the 800 pages of the NAS report.

Some 15 years have now passed since the NAS and MacLennan–Smith reports. Many more studies have been undertaken, and many more reports written. The massive NAS report has been updated every two years since 1994. In the light of new research there has been some adjustment in the allocation of diseases between the various categories, with four cancers now listed in the 'sufficient evidence' category and another four in the 'limited evidence' category.

One report of particular interest and relevance to our present concerns is *Cancer Incidence in Australian Vietnam Veterans*, published in 2005.[13] Based on evidence collected between 1982 and 2000 concerning the almost 60,000 Vietnam veterans, this report concluded that Australia's Vietnam veterans were at greater risk of cancer than the general community. But it also noted that the same was true of Australian Korean War veterans, suggesting that factors other than the herbicides that were deployed in Vietnam, but not in Korea, were at fault. Moreover, the most common form of cancer in the Vietnam veterans was melanoma, which has not been associated with herbicides. As indicated in Table 7-1 of this report (see Table 1), the association

Table 1
Herbicide related cancers in Australian Vietnam veterans

Disease	NAS Category	Result in this study
Chronic Lymphoid Leukaemia	Sufficient	Significantly elevated
Soft Tissue Sarcoma	Sufficient	Does not differ from expectation
Non Hodgkin's Lymphoma	Sufficient	Significantly decreased
Hodgkin's Disease	Sufficient	Significantly elevated
Lung Cancer	Limited	Significantly elevated
Prostate Cancer	Limited	Significantly elevated
Multiple Myeloma	Limited	Significantly decreased
Larynx Cancer	Limited	Significantly elevated

From E.J. Wilson, K.W. Horsley, R. van der Hoek, *Cancer Incidence in Australian Vietnam Veterans*, Department of Veterans' Affairs, Canberra, 2005, Table 7.1 (reproduced with permission of the Department of Veterans' Affairs).

between Australian Vietnam veterans and the cancers now listed in the top two categories of the NAS report is notably inconsistent. Of the four in the 'sufficient' category, two show a significantly elevated risk for veterans, one a significantly decreased risk, and the fourth is right on the community level. Of the four in the 'limited evidence' category, three show a significantly elevated risk, but the fourth a significantly decreased risk.

The discussion in the report concludes, with the uncertainty that characterises so many such reports, that the reasons for this variation, and the reasons for the overall levels of cancer, are 'unclear'. It notes the possibility that the herbicides might be a contributing factor; but it also refers pointedly to the association of some of the more common cancers among veterans with two well-known human carcinogens – alcohol consumption and cigarette smoking. It also notes that another known human carcinogen, asbestos, was present in large quantities on the RAN ships which transported thousands of army and air force personnel to and from Vietnam.

The figures in Table C-1 of this study, including the absolute numbers of cases, are also of considerable relevance (see Table 2). The worst offenders are in the hundreds, while many others are in the tens. Hodgkin's disease, for example, is one of the cancers in the 'sufficient evidence' category with an elevated risk of disease; but we are talking about 51 sufferers against an expected 25. Compare these figures with the more than 16,500 Vietnam veterans who have one or more accepted disabilities that are psychological or related to mental health.[14] The report on *Cancer Incidence in Australian Vietnam Veterans*, again without asserting definite conclusions, refers pointedly to the known carcinogenic effects of the combination of combat stress and alcohol, as well as the combination of smoking and alcohol.

Furthermore, just recently has come news of a report by a team of University of Sydney scientists at the Anzac Research Institute at Concord Hospital.[15] It seems that Australian Vietnam veterans are presenting disproportionately high numbers of certain physical and mental ailments, and that the most likely causes come back to that familiar trio: combat stress, smoking and alcohol consumption. Even now, more than 40 years after the first battalion was committed to Vietnam, we are still learning more about the effects of that trio of malefactors, either solo or in combination. And they were precisely the matters to which the Evatt Royal Commission had drawn attention in the 1980s, receiving the commendation of F.B. Smith in the early 1990s.

This, I suggest, points to the real tragedy of the story. Vietnam veterans had every right, and their organisations the responsibility, to press for compensation for the diverse ailments that afflicted them in the decades after their war service. With the benefit of hindsight, we can only regret that the Agent Orange lobby, by insisting that Vietnam was different from other wars and that herbicides used in Vietnam were the dominant cause of a great range of postwar ailments, took the whole debate about compensation for Vietnam veterans into a blind alley.

While endless inquiries and reports were analysing the effects of herbicides, too little attention was being given too slowly to more important questions such as post-traumatic stress and the effects of smoking and alcohol, to which the Evatt Royal Commission and other major studies had pointed. It now seems likely that the herbicides may have made some contribution to some of the ailments from which the veterans suffered, but numerically they were far outweighed by those caused by stress, smoking and alcohol. The real breakthroughs in addressing postwar ailments have come in addressing those areas. Whatever its motives and intentions, the Agent Orange lobby distorted and delayed the way in which the great majority of ailing Vietnam veterans could be compensated.

From what I have written, it will be clear that I see no merit in withdrawing or rewriting Smith's essay, which stands up well in the light of later evidence. Nevertheless, I do believe there is a case for a new study of the Agent Orange story, and not least the Australian dimension. There is now much more to write about than was the case when Smith wrote in the early 1990s, including but not confined to the reports that I have just discussed. I would welcome a thorough and independent study by anyone who could write authoritatively about

Table 2

All Service branches, Vietnam veterans: Observed and expected number of cancers, and standardised incidence ratios (SIRs). Period examined: 1982–2000.

Cancer type	Observed	Scenario 1 (excluding veterans whose status is unknown)			Scenario 2 (including veterans whose status is unknown)		
		Expected	SIR	95% CI	Expected	SIR	95% CI
All cancers	4590	3977	1.15	1.12–1.19	4077	1.13	1.09–1.16
Brain	97	91	1.07	0.85–1.28	93	1.04	0.84–1.25
Breast	7	8	0.90	0.36–1.86	8	0.88	0.35–1.81
Connective soft tissue	35	36	0.99	0.66–1.31	36	0.96	0.64–1.28
Eye	27	15	1.75	1.09–2.41	16	1.71	1.06–2.35
Gastrointestinal	743	710	1.05	0.97–1.12	727	1.02	0.95–1.09
Colorectal	622	580	1.07	0.99–1.16	594	1.05	0.96–1.13
Colon	376	334	1.13	1.01–1.24	342	1.10	0.99–1.21
Rectum	234	236	0.99	0.86–1.12	242	0.97	0.84–1.09
Stomach	104	116	0.89	0.72–1.07	119	0.87	0.70–1.04
Genitourinary	1055	922	1.14	1.08–1.21	947	1.11	1.05–1.18
Bladder	164	157	1.04	0.88–1.20	161	1.02	0.86–1.17
Kidney	125	124	1.01	0.83–1.19	127	0.99	0.81–1.16
Prostate	692	553	1.25	1.16–1.34	570	1.21	1.12–1.31
Testis	54	62	0.87	0.63–1.10	64	0.85	0.62–1.07
Hodgkin's disease	51	25	2.05	1.49–2.61	25	2.01	1.45–2.56
Leukaemia	130	110	1.18	0.98–1.38	113	1.15	0.95–1.35
Lymphoid leukaemia	72	52	1.38	1.06–1.69	54	1.34	1.03–1.65

LL acute	9	7	1.29	0.59–2.44	7	1.26	0.58–2.39
LL chronic	58	37	1.55	1.15–1.95	38	1.51	1.12–1.90
Myeloid leukaemia	54	52	1.03	0.75–1.30	54	1.00	0.74–1.27
ML acute	30	29	1.04	0.67–1.42	29	1.02	0.65–1.38
ML chronic	21	17	1.20	0.69–1.71	18	1.17	0.67–1.67
Liver	27	38	0.70	0.44–0.97	39	0.69	0.43–0.95
Lung	576	468	1.23	1.13–1.33	480	1.20	1.10–1.30
Adenocarcinoma	188	130	1.45	1.24–1.66	133	1.41	1.21–1.62
Squamous	152	127	1.19	1.00–1.38	131	1.16	0.98–1.35
Small-cell	87	71	1.23	0.97–1.49	73	1.20	0.95–1.45
Large-cell	79	74	1.07	0.83–1.31	76	1.04	0.81–1.27
Other	70	66	1.06	0.81–1.30	68	1.03	0.79–1.27
Melanoma	756	573	1.32	1.23–1.41	586	1.29	1.20–1.38
Mesothelioma	27	34	0.81	0.50–1.11	34	0.79	0.49–1.08
Multiple myeloma	31	47	0.66	0.43–0.90	48	0.65	0.42–0.88
NHL	126	189	0.67	0.55–0.79	193	0.65	0.54–0.77
Oesophagus	70	57	1.22	0.94–1.51	59	1.19	0.91–1.47
Oral cavity, pharynx, larynx	344	233	1.47	1.32–1.63	239	1.44	1.29–1.59
Head and neck	247	167	1.48	1.29–1.66	171	1.44	1.26–1.63
Larynx	97	66	1.46	1.17–1.75	68	1.43	1.14–1.71
Pancreas	86	75	1.15	0.91–1.40	77	1.12	0.89–1.36
Thyroid	17	30	0.57	0.33–0.92	30	0.56	0.33–0.90
Unknown	143	135	1.06	0.89–1.24	138	1.04	0.87–1.21

From E.J. Wilson, K.W. Horsley, R. van der Hoek, *Cancer Incidence in Australian Vietnam Veterans*, Department of Veterans' Affairs, Canberra, 2005, Table C.1 (reproduced with permission of the Department of Veterans' Affairs).

the attitudes and actions of veterans and veterans' organisations, of elected politicians and their official advisers, of medical and biological scientists, of statisticians, of lawyers and of workers in the media. My personal expectation, based on the matters discussed in this paper, is that a new account by such an author or authors might possibly temper one or two of Smith's more caustic judgements on individuals, but that overall he or she or they would applaud Smith's account and endorse its major themes. In particular, a new account would probably reflect Smith's succinct summary, that Australia's Agent Orange story is 'a tangle of decency and folly, of courage and chicanery, but above all waste'.

A short walk in a minefield

Tony White

February 1967 was the worst month for casualties for the Australian Task Force in the Vietnam War up to that point. That record stood for some time to come. The 5th Battalion, Royal Australian Regiment (5RAR), was by then nine months into its first tour of duty.

On 21 February 1967 an infantry patrol of 5RAR's B Company, mounted on armoured personnel carriers (APCs), ran into a minefield. This incident caused 35 of the 73 casualties sustained by the Task Force that month.

The battalion was tasked with a week-long search-and-destroy operation – Operation Renmark – on the eastern side of the Long Hai hills which lay on the coast of South Vietnam's Phuoc Tuy province.

The hills had been a guerrilla haven since French colonial times and were known to the National Liberation Front as the Minh Dam Secret Zone. Rising to 330 metres, they were riddled with caves containing extensive Viet Cong facilities. Earlier that February, during Tet, the lunar New Year festival, a Viet Cong flag, spot-lit at night, flew defiantly from a flagpole at the southern end of the hills. Eight months earlier, the US 173d Airborne Brigade had conducted a sweep through the area, suffering heavy casualties.

The lead-up to Operation Renmark was not propitious. A week

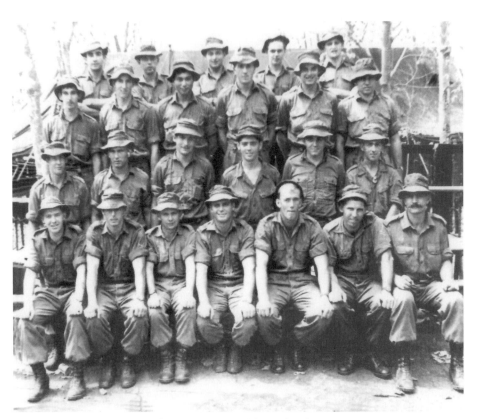

The human cost of mine warfare. Australian soldiers of 4 Platoon, B Company, 5RAR, at the task force base, Nui Dat, South Vietnam, January 1967. On 21 February, 4 Platoon suffered severe casualties in a dual mine incident while patrolling near the Long Hai hills. Seven Australians were killed and 28 were wounded, two of whom also later died. Popular leader Lieutenant Jack Carruthers, who died from his wounds, is at the right end of the front row. (Image courtesy of Tony White.)

earlier, the battalion's C Company suffered grievously in a booby trap incident that resulted in eight casualties, including the deaths of three officers. The day before the planned start, our sister battalion, 6RAR, was caught in a ferocious firefight (Operation Bribie) close by; this delayed our start and denied us the element of surprise. Nevertheless, the first two days of the search were comparatively uneventful. On the third day, the companies moved south to position themselves for the second phase of the operation.

At 1.30 pm on 21 February, B Company, mounted on APCs, set forth towards the base of the hills. Battalion headquarters, with whom I was travelling, was to follow after half an hour. Just as we were preparing to depart, we heard a loud explosion and saw a black mushroom cloud rising above the trees in B Company's line of travel. Four minutes later there was a second smaller explosion and a cloud of dust. A radio call soon followed requesting a 'dust-off', the code for a helicopter casualty evacuation. Details were sketchy, but clearly the patrol had struck a minefield and there were heavy casualties.

By chance a two-man Bell reconnaissance helicopter was at our battalion headquarters position, and I was soon on my way to the scene, just two kilometres away. As we banked to find a suitable spot to land, we saw an incredible sight: an APC was lying over on its side, its track blown off; soldiers and equipment lay scattered over an area the size of a tennis court. The pilot dropped me off in a tiny clearing close by. As the clatter of the departing helicopter faded, I was struck by the silence of the hot, dry, dusty patch of bush. There were groans and mutterings of the wounded, but no screams or hysteria. Most of the troops were just stunned.

I was met by Ron Nichols, B Company's medical corps corporal, and Jock Bouse, the stretcher-bearer corporal. Both had been wounded. We set to work. The first group of casualties I encountered were those of B Company's headquarters. The company commander, Major Bruce McQualter, had a head wound. He was conscious, struggling to stand up, but unable to respond to questions or commands. Stretched out next to him, also with a head wound and unconscious, was the commander of 4 Platoon, Lieutenant Jack Carruthers. The platoon sergeant, Tassie Wass, was the most urgent casualty with both elbows shattered and wounds to the back. I made him comfortable with morphine and applied dressings to his wounds.

Near the back of the upturned APC there was a pyramid of what at first glance appeared to be discarded equipment and uniforms. It was dark gray in colour. On closer inspection it proved to be a pile of dead and wounded soldiers blown out of the back of the APC. It was not until 30 years later that I discovered the cause of the blackened skin and uniforms. Two layers of sandbags had been laid on the floor of the APCs as protection against mines. The sand used was very fine and black; the boys had literally been sandblasted by the explosion.

Many of the wounded were suffering from the effects of the

War Wounds

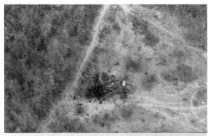

An aerial view of the site, two months after the mine incident on 21 February 1967 (refer to sketch below). The burnt hull of the destroyed armoured personnel carrier lies abandoned and the deep crater of the anti-tank mine detonation is still visible.
(AWM P06362.012)

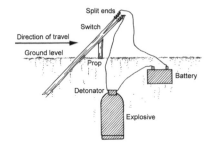

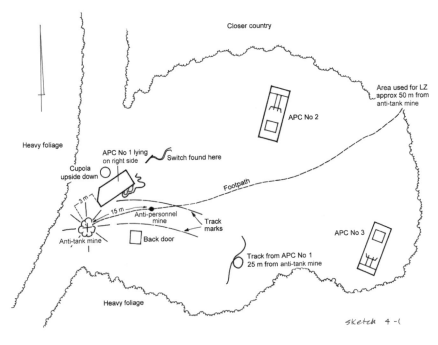

The site of the mine incident on 21 February 1967, when an armoured personnel carrier detonated a Viet Cong anti-tank mine fabricated from an American 5-inch naval shell and a simple but effective firing switch (inset top left). The explosion killed five soldiers and wounded nine others. Minutes later, soldiers rushing to their aid detonated a Viet Cong-laid anti-personnel mine which killed two more men and wounded 19 others. Battalion RMO, Captain Tony White, confronted a scene of carnage as he flew in by helicopter to assist. (Sketch reproduced from Ian McNeill and Ashley Ekins, *On the Offensive*, 2003, p. 118.)

explosive blast and were peppered with shrapnel. They required little treatment apart from shell dressings and lots of reassurance. On the other hand, there were some horrific sights, including an arm and hand grasping a rifle and protruding from under the APC, the soldier having been crushed to death. There was a torso of another soldier separated by some distance from the lower half of his body.

Of the 35 casualties, seven were killed. Soon dust-off helicopters started arriving. It was a busy time, trying to get casualties away in order of need. The last casualties were evacuated within 90 minutes of the explosions. Over the next few days two of the wounded, Major McQualter and Lieutenant Jack Carruthers, died in hospital of their head wounds.

So what had caused this catastrophe? The engineers did a thorough forensic job in piecing together what had happened. The convoy's lead APC had been hit by a buried explosive of immense power, resulting in a crater nearly two metres across and one metre deep. The 11-tonne vehicle was thrown three metres away, landing on its side. Fortunately for those riding inside, the back door was blown off. One of the APC tracks was sent flying over the top of the second vehicle, landing about ten metres back. The APC driver and commander and three soldiers were killed. Nine others were wounded.

The explosive was a recycled 5-inch US Navy shell. It had a simple switch made of copper wire wound around the ends of a length of split bamboo. Pressure from a passing vehicle squeezed the split ends together, completing the electrical circuit and detonating the bomb. Extremely economical, this was a classic bit of guerrilla recycling.[1]

Major McQualter and his party moved forward to render aid to the casualties. But then disaster struck once again. One of McQualter's party stepped on an M16 mine, killing another two soldiers and wounding 19. The distance between the two explosions was 15 metres. Some of the soldiers wounded in the first blast were wounded a second time by the M16 mine, which contained half a kilo of TNT. When a downward force was applied to the pressure prongs – typically from a soldier's boot – a charge was set off propelling the mine about a metre above ground, where it exploded. It had a lethal radius of about 25 metres.

These mines were known as 'Jumping Jacks'. They would continue to cause a huge proportion of Australian casualties for the rest of the war. To add insult to injury, they were all lifted by the enemy from minefields around the posts of our allies and, later, from our own notorious 'barrier minefield'.

So what should be done when a patrol runs into a minefield and sustains casualties? Common sense says that everyone should freeze until the sappers get in and clear the area. Helpers can endanger themselves and others by triggering off further mines – exactly as happened here.

Corporal Bluey Bryant swears to this day that a fellow section commander shouted at me to stop (else he would shoot me) as I walked in after being dropped off by the helicopter. I have no recollection of this, but am grateful that he failed to act on his warning. The sappers arrived with their mine-detecting gear about 20 minutes after the blasts. Even though the two medics and I had been busy around the area well before mine-clearing got under way, I nevertheless received a sound bollocking from one of the sappers for not sticking to their cleared area.

After this incident, it became standard procedure for all person-nel to freeze until the area was cleared by sappers. This must have presented some agonising dilemmas. Soldiers had to curb their instinct to go to the aid of a comrade who might have been only metres away, but in pain or bleeding to death.

What were my own feelings during the course of that afternoon? I experienced a chaotic succession of emotions. During my year in Vietnam, I found the hardest time of all was from that moment of being despatched to attend to casualties until my arrival on the scene. What would I have to deal with? One had no idea what was in store except that it would invariably be awful. Would I be overwhelmed? Would I be up to it? This anxiety far outweighed any fear of being killed or wounded. Naively, I believed the Diggers wouldn't let that happen to *their* Doc. Still it was in a fever of anxiety and apprehension that I flew into the location of the disaster. On arriving, the anxiety was quickly supplanted by horror and disbelief. I couldn't believe what I was seeing and hearing. After a year with the battalion, I knew many of the Diggers quite well; these dead and wounded soldiers were not strangers.

The scale of the task was almost crushing. Every step revealed some fresh awfulness. The horror and disbelief now gave way to sheer terror – knowing that we were stalled in a minefield and that I could go the way of those I was trying to help. One thing I'll never forget was looking down and seeing the three prongs of an M16 protruding from the dust, only inches from my boot heel. My mind was a whirlwind of wild racing thoughts – snippets of memories of home and family, old movies, anatomy lessons – all, no doubt, some desperate protection against blind panic.

Finally came profound relief after the sappers had done their job and the last casualties were on their way. But I was a shaken wreck.

I've often been asked, 'What did you do?' My answer, 'Not a lot!', might sound a bit disingenuous, but it is true. This was First Aid – which doesn't call for a medical degree. In Vietnam we were very fortunate in having a superb aero-medical evacuation system that had some casualties on the operating table in hospital within 30 minutes of being wounded. Deciding on priorities for evacuation was important.

A lot of the wounded were just severely bruised and concussed by the explosions. Morphine was administered to those in pain using syrettes. These were collapsible tubes like a miniature toothpaste tube with an attached needle. Controlling bleeding was obviously top of the list, and we used a lot of shell dressings. These were thick gauze pads with attached ribbons with which they could be tied over the wound. They contained a glass ampoule, which was smashed to saturate the wound and dressing with iodine. The packs bore a date stamp showing that they had been manufactured in England in April 1915, the month of the ANZAC landings on Gallipoli. Over half a century later, they were still perfectly serviceable: I still keep one as a souvenir.

Simply being there and offering comfort was the best medicine.

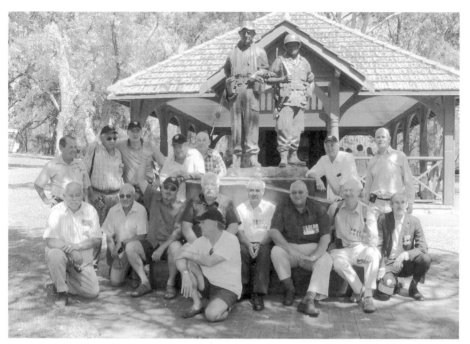

Veterans of 4 Platoon, B Company, 5RAR, including survivors of the mine incident in the Long Hai hills, gather for a reunion in Perth in 2007. Former RMO Dr Tony White is at the right end of the back row. (Image courtesy of Tony White.)

Many a Digger involved in this and other casualty situations has remarked on how reassured he was to see the Doc arrive on the scene.

The battalion medics often fretted about how they'd handled this or that casualty, especially under pressure. I'd reassure them, saying that, of course, we'd all do things better the second time around: you just do the best you can. I do not believe that the two soldiers who died in hospital of their head wounds from this incident in the minefield could have been saved by first aid in the field.

Every two years the boys of 4 Platoon, now in their sixties, and their families meet for a reunion. I am honoured to be invited to join them. How are they doing? Overall – and not surprisingly – not that well. Physically, most of them, at the very least, have back or leg problems. Psychologically, most were damaged to some degree by this catastrophic event in their young lives. But with time the reunions are, if anything, becoming a lot more cheerful and upbeat. There's no whinging and whining; they're getting on with life. I salute them.

Military nursing in Afghanistan, 2008

Sharon Cooper[1]

Of the many war memorials in this country, one with the greatest significance is the Australian Service Nurses National Memorial, which stands on ANZAC Parade in Canberra. It commemorates Australia's nurses and honours those who have served and suffered in conflict. The diary extracts of past service nurses, transcribed on the memorial in a style that replicates their own handwriting, provide us with a unique insight into the reality of their experience of war. Some panels of the memorial, intentionally left blank, also remind us of those who continue to serve today and those who will serve in the future.

Australian service nurses have exhibited great courage and sacrifice in every major military operation in which Australia has been involved: one might recall the seven Australian nurses who were awarded Military Medals for bravery under fire on the Western Front, those who gave their lives in the Banka Island massacre and the sinking of the hospital ship *Centaur* during the Second World War, and more recently, the horrific Sea King helicopter crash in Indonesia in 2005.

Since 2004, six Australian Defence Force (ADF) critical care teams have been deployed to war – three to Iraq and three to Afghanistan.

All six were commanded by nurses. In 2008 I became one of these nurses entrusted with command in a theatre of war.

As a nurse, I could provide a great deal of clinical detail concerning the wounds of war, but instead, in the spirit of the diary extracts on the walls of the Australian Service Nurses National Memorial, I would like to share with readers my personal experience of service. I hope that this will allow you to reflect on what today's wounds of war might be, by seeing how I described some of them in the fragmentary diary I kept throughout my service, most recently during my time in Afghanistan.

I begin with my very first entries of my Afghanistan journal:

A Tuesday in July
Departure.

A Wednesday in July
Arrival.

A Thursday in July
I already feel incredibly attached to my team, and I think I catch glimpses of their attachment to me. I don't want to disappoint them or fail them but I struggle with the knowledge that I cannot protect them from their personal experience of this journey. I can't protect them. I can't deliver them home to their families in the condition I received them. They are already changed. Oddly I continue to not have any concern for my own welfare. I accept that I will be changed and hope that the positives outweigh the alternatives. I must continue to concentrate on the positives of this adventure in order to bring my people home better for having been with me.

This certainty that the experience of war would change me and my team came from my own previous experiences of active service. I was first exposed to the sacrifices of service early in my career, in

February 2000, when I was posted as an operating theatre nurse to East Timor. During my six-month deployment on this peacekeeping operation, six United Nations peacekeepers of varied military uniforms, including Australians and New Zealanders, lost their lives in the service of their countries, and in the service of East Timor. While only one of these deaths occurred in direct combat with an opposing force, all occurred on foreign soil far from their family and loved ones. Here for the first time – within only 12 months of having enlisted – I began to appreciate exactly what I had signed up for: to protect and preserve, with compassion and with skill, but mostly with courage.

Four years later I returned to East Timor to learn my next valuable lesson in the wounds of war: on 2 June 2004 I boarded a helicopter as an aero-medical evacuation nurse to fly to the aid of an East Timorese woman whose life was threatened by the obstructed labour that had already claimed the life of her unborn child.

The mood was friendly and jovial as we rose into the sky above Dili, and my thoughts quickly turned to the patient we had been called to evacuate. We were headed to the village of Same, on the other side of a mountain range which was rapidly becoming shrouded by stormy weather. Our final approach into the village revealed a break in cloud cover to reveal the ground and a river bed. The pilots agreed to attempt to follow the river bed. The rain became heavier, decreasing visibility through the front windscreen. The rescue crewman opened the right hand door to aid his visibility of the ground, allowing the pelting rain to stream in.

I was still not concerned for my own safety. I was aware that the crew were working very hard and I had considered that we simply may not reach Same that day. I worried about the patient whose life may be depending upon our arrival.

Then I heard the pilot's alarming words.

'We're going in! Brace, brace, brace!'

We're what? Through the front windscreen I could now see

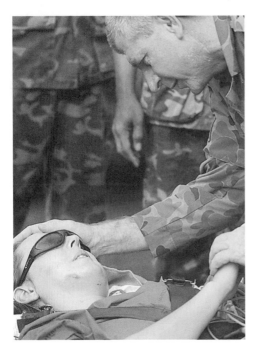

Flight Lieutenant Sharon Cooper being comforted by Lieutenant Colonel Ross Bradford after she survived a helicopter crash in June 2004 while serving with the United Nations support mission in East Timor. Suffering a broken back and broken jaw, she was repatriated to Australia and began the long and painful task of learning to walk again.
(Image courtesy of Private John Wellfare, Department of Defence.)

that we were racing toward the trees. The visibility was suddenly clear and we were flying toward the ground. I instinctively lent forward, crossed my arms across the front of my shins and grabbed my ankles. I looked to my right to observe the doctor assuming the same position. His actions mirrored my own and assured me that this was really happening.

'Mayday, mayday . . . '

This was it. So sudden. So surreal. So powerless to alter the rapid change of course my life was about to take. A course which may well be the end. The crew frantically followed their drills as we sat motionless, waiting, helpless. I gripped my ankles and held myself firm as the world rushed past me. My life didn't flash before my eyes, but in an instant, almost subconsciously, I accounted for my loved ones and knew that they would all survive this, only my partner would be left alone. My last feelings were of fear for my life intermingled with sorrow. I quietly apologised to him and my world fell silent.

Then, pain ripped through my body. The mechanical whir of the transmission accentuated the fearful smell of fuel and I realised that we had only just hit the ground. I was alive and I had to get out.

We had crashed but I was alive. My back and left hip hurt, my left leg refused to move. I could taste blood as my tongue located my lower left jaw in the centre of my mouth. The aroma of aviation fuel permeated the world and my flying suit was wet with it, as the searing cold pain of the fuel began to corrode my skin.

The wounds I received that day were acutely visible at the time to my colleagues, friends and family. You may think that our external wounds are more visible than any of the emotional or psychological ones we receive, but no one can see the serious spinal fracture that I will carry for the remainder of my life, nor the multiple plates and screws which, although now redundant, served their purpose in mending my fractured jaw. The physical wounds of war, however, will not always be clearly visible, nor do they need to be. I have worked hard to cover my wounds, not to be defined by my injuries or that single moment in my life; and daily, as a serving member, I continue to strive to prove my value to my service despite my injuries.

Just recently, a friend of mine who is a veteran of Rwanda explained to a polite enquirer, 'No matter where you go in this job, you always leave a piece of yourself there.' I am sure that he had spent many years reflecting upon his period of service, and he had summed up a sense of what I had always thought about my own service, but had never been adequately able to express in words. I have a strong affection for East Timor, even feel a personal bond with this, the place in which arguably my most dramatic wounds were received. I could be flippant and say that I earned my best war story there. I could also be melodramatic and say that it is because my blood was spilt there. But while that fact certainly resonates with me, I prefer to look a little deeper and acknowledge that it was in the service of this fledgling country that I learnt the true value of life – and, in particular, of my own. The small piece of myself that I left behind was indeed my innocence.

While this inevitable change to oneself that comes with service may reflect a type of wounding, a loss of something, there can also

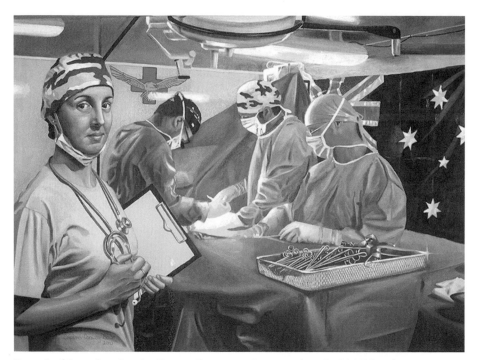

Portrait of Squadron Leader Sharon Cooper as Commander of a RAAF Combat Surgical Team in Afghanistan in 2008, painted by her husband Captain Conway Bown.
(Image courtesy of Squadron Leader Sharon Bown.)

be powerful gains; I certainly have never felt as alive as during my service in Afghanistan. There I was working to my absolute maximum physically, emotionally, intellectually, spiritually. The patients presenting in need of our care required life- or limb-saving intervention. The coughs and colds of home gave way to massive haemorrhage and the gross disfigurement of traumatic amputations, stabbings, gunshot, blast injury and the devastating impact of the improvised explosive devices which tore through young, vital human flesh with such ease. I was required to draw upon every aspect of my clinical and military training. I began to feel more like a military officer than I ever had before. I had nursed before, I had deployed before, but I had never been to war before. In my life before Afghanistan, this kind of scene would have felt like a Hollywood creation. As clichéd as it might sound, in quiet moments I would find myself humming the theme from *MASH*, but in the face of reality and the heat of action, it was all too real.

A Monday in August

Big trauma day. Biggest so far. Up from 0600 until 0300 with only two very short sit-down meals for rest.

First patient – X 1 Local National Policeman. Execution type gun shot wounds x 3. Entry wound with burn to R cheek, exit wound tore open left corner of mouth across left cheek. L[eft] shoulder flesh wound. Entry L side of larynx, came to rest posterior to C5-6 resulting in unstable fracture and tetraplegia. Prognosis very poor, although fracture stabilised with Miami soft collar and wounds debrided and closed. My doctors, having done all that they can, have shown such sensitivity to this man and his family, explaining that there is nothing more that can be done. I watch the pain and remorse on their faces. The patient was so annoyed with them. Not because of the news that they were delivering, but because the time that they were taking to do so was interfering with his enjoyment of fresh fruit being fed to him by the nurses. Inshallah, if it be God's will. This will not be the last time I witness [people of] this culture accept their fate so willingly, and as a result be able to savour precisely what they have at that moment in time. With my upbringing I ponder how lucky I have been to be born in Australia. If I ever feel annoyed to be waiting for healthcare, I hope that I remember Sardar and his four children, who will grow up in this desperate place without him. I hope that I also remember to appreciate the small time that I have while I have it.

Second patient – X 1 Local National. Gunshot wound x 2, chest and L[eft] thigh. Flesh wounds only. Very lucky, good prognosis. Not keen to talk, or even to give us a name. Whose side is he on? There are no distinguishing marks or features and even if there were, I hope that his existence as a human being will always override his actions and beliefs when we as Australians deliver him healthcare.

Third and final patient – X 1 NATO soldier with traumatic amputations of both hands. Apparently he was adjusting a grenade on his belt, behind his back, when it exploded. An accident. The ends of his arms are unrecognisable – shredded flesh, yet the remainder of his body is untouched, protected by his body armour. I'm torn between thinking his luck today has been good and yet [it was] so bad. One of my surgeons later tells me that in his phone call home to his wife, he expressed just how lucky he is to be alive to be able to continue to love her and to love their baby. It dawns on me that I am the lucky one today for having had the honour to meet him, to help him, and to learn from him.

Despite the immense tragedy of this persistent parade of combat trauma suffered by combatants, I found that I could preserve my sanity and accept my own duty in this war. But it meant altering my perspective: I could accept that these men had, for whatever reason, taken up arms in this conflict. They had made a choice of sorts, whether good or bad, to be here in this war. Some had even taken up arms in an attempt to resolve domestic disputes completely unrelated to the conflict around them. The patients who really challenged my resilience, however, were the children (and it is with their fates that I continue to struggle). I had never dealt with paediatric trauma before, and while the children we saw in Afghanistan were not wounded as a direct result of combatant activity, they were victims of a society at war, a society that was struggling to protect them. Of those that I saw, they truly seemed to be the innocent victims.

A Friday in August

How does an eight-year-old boy get shot with a hand gun at 0500 hrs in the morning in his family home? I will never forget the feel of his chest under my hands as I levered my body up and down to pump his heart. Nor the colour that drained from him when after an hour of pumping and willing his heart to restart, we as a team decided that we could do no more to bring him back to us. A child that cried for someone or something in his mother's tongue as we put him to sleep, cried to a room full of strangers who could not understand his pleas. Where was his mother? Why does her culture prevent her from being beside her child as he fights for his life?

Of course, it was not just the children of Afghanistan who fought for their lives far from their families: there were also our Australian soldiers. Once again, eight years after first confronting the loss of one who wore my uniform, I was honoured to be there when those who were risking their lives in the service of their country now desperately needed to be cared for themselves.

A Tuesday in September

We receive the largest number of Australian combat casualties in one attack since the Vietnam War. It is not at all surprising that my team did a magnificent job, and although I know that having Aussies come through the trauma doors tugged at their heart strings, they conducted themselves with the utmost professionalism, compassion and good old Aussie mateship. My heart swells with pride to think of their actions on this night. There is little more confronting than treating one who wears your uniform. I ask myself how I return home, how I return my team home, if we leave one of our own behind. As we worked with our Australian casualties I made a concerted effort to remember the Christian names of each of the boys as we treated them so that when I spoke to their mates and Commanders throughout the night I hoped that I could convey that they were as important to us as they were to them, and that there was absolutely no chance that we would leave them behind.

A Thursday in September

Today I had the honour of again caring for one of our own. A battle-weary Australian soldier, who, from the adrenaline-fuelled anecdotes of the trauma room, [I knew] had fought against other men to preserve the life of the mates that fought beside him and to save himself. He was tired. He was dirty. His injuries were such that he would not return to the battlefield before first returning home. As his anaesthetic faded, he opened his eyes. He looked at me, and with the courtesy of a true gentleman, a tempered soldier, he said three words. 'Thank you Ma'am.' There I was in awe of what he was prepared to do for his country, for the country of strangers who could be friend or foe, while I secured myself and my team behind the defences – and he was thanking me. In one moment and three words, every hardship of this and every other aspect of my military life disappeared. If I achieved nothing more in my years of service than aiding in the safe return of this soldier, it was possible that I had done enough.

I am but one member of the ADF, and my stories make up just one subset of a far greater whole. The wounds of war are far more intractable and go far deeper in our nation than perhaps we care to acknowledge, but let that not cast a shadow on our service. Australian service nurses have consistently exhibited great courage and sacrifice in every major military operation in which the nation has been involved. Not only have they tended the wounds of war, they have themselves also suffered from such wounds and survived them. Through their actions, Australian service nurses reveal that although conflict and war demonstrate the very worst of humanity, they often also reveal the very best.

So as you pause to commemorate, recognise and reflect upon the sacrifice and service of all Australians in all areas and ages of conflict, remember as well those who have pledged to continue to serve. Remember those who are separated from home and loved ones in a foreign land in the service of their country. Think too of those who are ready without hesitation to walk away from their lives in the service of others; think of my colleagues who will kiss their children goodbye in the dark of night, not knowing if and when they might see them again – just so they can do their part to prepare for them a better, more just world. Think of those who simply love what they do. Despite the wounds of war, I am proud to be one of you.

Living with war wounds

Graham Edwards

In writing this chapter, I have had to reflect deeply on many memories over a 40-year period. It has been an interesting journey to delve back into the far recesses of my mind and disturb the coffins long interred and nailed shut. Some were memories perhaps better left buried.

Life post-Vietnam was a rollercoaster ride of emotions: joy, sadness, hope, despair, laughter, tears, achievement, failure, peace, turmoil, pain, loneliness, and anger. All of these emotions were underpinned by being a young man grateful to have survived a war, but one who thought often of what might have been as he battled to come to grips with what was and what is. Determined but uncertain. Outwardly confident, but privately fragile and pained. Many of these emotions were experienced in a time and an environment where Vietnam veterans were returning to the cold shoulder of indifference, ignorance, even hostility.

Like many Vietnam veterans I have now grown used to not thinking of Vietnam for weeks but then thinking of nothing else for days.

I recall with great clarity the mine incident which should have killed me, but didn't. I recall sitting in the red dirt, watching it turned to mud by my spilled blood. Looking at my shattered legs. Clutching

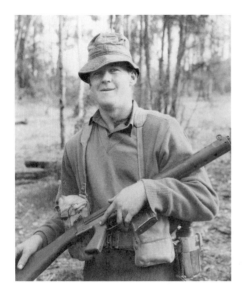

Private Graham Edwards of 7RAR, during a training exercise in Australia in 1969 shortly before he departed for a tour of duty in South Vietnam. Edwards had been 'in country' for four months when he was severely wounded by an M16 anti-personnel mine explosion that resulted in the amputation of his legs. (AWM P04724.001)

my machine-gun, afraid to put it down in case it triggered another mine. Repeating to myself, with great intensity: 'I am not going to die; I am not going to die.'

Listening to my mates, frantic to get to me with first aid but knowing that they had to be disciplined, cautious, and patient. The whole time experiencing incredible and indescribable pain, which broke over me in agonising waves. Being tormented by the sound of the CO's Bell helicopter as it darted and twisted in the safety above. His not sharing the danger of those he commanded below. Listening for the sweet and comforting sound of the dust-off chopper that I knew would be in the air within minutes of the mine explosion.

I had been wounded some weeks before and pulled out of the jungle in the dark of night and whisked to 1 Australian Field Hospital, where I was treated by very professional and competent medical people. I drew great comfort from that previous experience and knew that neither the hospital team nor my mates on the ground, working frantically and with great courage to get to me, would let me down.

I was conscious right till the time they wheeled me from triage into the operating theatre, and as they put me under the anaesthetic, I remember looking into the eyes of the surgeon as he studied my X-rays and feeling sorry for him.

When I awoke the next morning, I knew my legs were gone and it was a matter of looking down to see how high the amputations were.

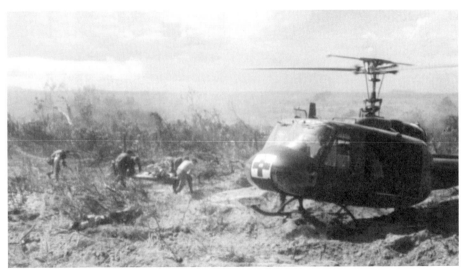

Private Graham Edwards is rushed to a 'dust-off' helicopter following his severe wounding in a mine explosion on 12 May 1970 near the Long Hai hills, Phuoc Tuy province, South Vietnam. (Image courtesy of Graham Edwards.)

Sitting by my bed was one of the surgeons who had operated. I might rue the loss of my legs later, but at that moment I was just elated to still be alive.

A couple of years ago I had the opportunity to speak at the national reunion of 1 Australian Field Hospital, and I used the opportunity to express eternal gratitude and appreciation for the job they did. They were one of the great Australian units that served in Vietnam, and their professionalism, skill, compassion, and care made a big difference to me and to many other wounded soldiers.

I recall when the time came for me to go home. One of the hardest things I ever experienced was saying goodbye to my close-knit mates, who came down to Vung Tau to say farewell. I felt like I was deserting them, and it was hard to hide the tears as we parted. The journey home was a long one, as I was taken off the plane at Butterworth air base in Malaysia and held there for a further two weeks. Though I hated it at the time, it was a good move as it enabled me to be stabilised medically and helped me to get a grip on my feelings.

We were 'snuck' back into Australia in the dead hours of the pre-dawn night. No welcome, no warmth, just an arrival designed to hide the flotsam and jetsam of wounded and ill soldiers returning from an unpopular war.

The next day I was transferred to Heidelberg hospital in Melbourne. All of the medical advice was that Heidelberg was the best hospital for me to go to. It was good advice.

The reunion with my wife Noelene and my seven-month-old daughter was an emotional one and it was good to feel the warmth of a family's embrace. They had been living with Noelene's family in Ballarat while I was in Vietnam.

I remember some time before I went overseas watching a soldier who had lost the lower part of his leg in Vietnam swimming at the pool at Holdsworthy army base. I thought then I would rather come home in a box than come home disabled. How wrong I was. I was just happy to be home alive, and grateful to have survived.

I had accepted the loss of my legs. Learning to live with the loss, however, would be a different matter. Having cheated death, I now had to learn to have a fulfilling life.

I was keen to get out of hospital, and six weeks after the mine incident, we moved into a flat not far from the hospital. Thus began my period of rehabilitation. When I look back, I remember that all I wanted to do was to be like any other husband and father, and provide security, a home, and a future for my family.

As a young bloke, I had hated school because all it taught me were the things I was not good at. I lived for footy and cricket and spent many a wagged day on the beach at Scarborough bodysurfing. I had left school the year I turned 15, never for one moment thinking that I would ever be out of work or need to rely on an education rather than a manual approach to employment. But I was about to pay the price for the neglect of my years at school.

I should also explain that my father had been badly knocked around during the Second World War. I remember countless weekends as a child visiting him at Hollywood 'repat' hospital in Perth. On one occasion after he'd had a long spell in hospital, the War Service Homes Commission wrote to him and told him that if he did not do something about the peeling paint on the outside of our home, they would take action. He had himself discharged from hospital, came home, and erected ladders and planks. And with his leg in plaster, he painted the outside of the house.

On discharge, he could not get a job and 'the repat' would not give him a 'T & PI' (Totally and Permanently Incapacitated) pension. He lost his business through his war-caused illness. But he was a tough bugger, my dad, and went back to his pre-war occupation as a miner and prospector. With some borrowed money and on the prospector's allowance he went bush with a pick strapped to one crutch and a shovel to the other.

It was not until I was older that I understood his suffering and just how hard 'repat' had been on him. The irony was that he made some good discoveries and pocketed a good few dollars – and no sooner had he got back on his feet than 'repat' gave him his 'T & PI'.

I was determined that they would not treat me as they had treated my father. But I still came under the charge of the army, and so I felt I had no option but to trust myself to the system; indeed, put my whole faith in it.

And so began my period of rehabilitation – the worst and most demeaning time of my life. I was fitted with artificial legs, and every morning I was picked up in a taxi and, along with others, taken to a former mansion in Toorak which served as a 'rehab' centre. I discovered it was a place for young people with learning difficulties. There I was joined by another 7th Battalion bloke, Sergeant Tom Bourke, who had also become an amputee following a mine incident.

My first session was 'physio', run by a woman drawn from 'the blue-rinse set'. Blue coiffured hair, painted nails, immaculate uniform. Her job was to assist me to learn to use my new legs. She excelled at chatter with her work mates, but showed no interest in her job. Every morning she simply said, 'Go for a walk.' The implication was that one shouldn't annoy her with tedious, job-related responsibilities.

The second period was 'O.T.' (Occupational Therapy): the task allocated to me was to make a breadboard. In the first week I was permitted to select a piece of wood and mark out the design of my board. In the second week I was allowed to cut a corner and sand it. At no time was I permitted to get ahead of the work schedule or timetable.

The third period was English, where I had to go to the back of the class, select a pre-determined book, read it, and answer multiple-choice questions: Who threw the ball? Did Dora throw the ball? Having finished the exercise, each student was to sit quietly in the class and not disturb the teacher.

Fourth period was maths. Here I excelled. Go to the back of the class, select the pre-determined book, and answer the multiple-choice questions $10 + 10 = ?$ Once finished, sit quietly, don't disturb the teacher.

Tom Bourke did his block and left. I couldn't blame him. However, I wanted to believe the system would come good, so was more patient. But I did go to the bloke who managed the facility and explained to him that this program was no good to me. He exploded, and accused me of not being grateful and not appreciating what my country was doing for me. He was indeed a great patriot.

Some things, however, did improve. But not 'physio', as 'Miss Hairdo' was still engrossed in last night's social function or the pile of women's magazines which weighed heavily on her desk.

'O.T.' improved as they allowed me to quickly finish the bread-board and then make a pair of moccasins. (I never have been able to fathom why they wanted a bloke with no feet to make himself a pair of moccasins.) Things in English and Maths also improved. I learnt that Dick caught the ball, and I was also allowed to explore the realms of simple long division.

I went to the Army and asked them to send me home to Western Australia. I think they were only too happy to do so. The Army in WA, however, was not so happy, as I found out later.

It was also a difficult time for my wife. Noelene came from a close-knit family who had grown to love their granddaughter. Dragging them off to the west was like taking them to a different country.

And so it was in many respects. When I alighted from the plane, my family went one way and I, despite vigorous argument, was ordered into an Army ambulance waiting on the tarmac. I was driven straight to the Army medical centre at Swanbourne, and it became evident that they wanted to admit me into hospital for assessment. It took strong argument to stop them.

It also became evident that the army wanted to discharge me without delay. In Victoria the Army had gone out of its way to find a job for Tom Bourke, with his rank of sergeant and his future secured. Within weeks in Perth, however, the Army had its way. It was 'sign here and bugger off'. It was a lonely feeling standing in the orderly room: no thanks, no legs, no 'Good onya, mate'. Just an uncertain future.

I had no option but to go back to school, and I wanted to sit for my Leaving or Year 12 certificate. But the education authorities would not allow it and demanded that I sit for my Junior (Year 10) certificate first. So it was back to study, and at the end of the year I sat my Junior.

Next year I enrolled at Leederville Technical College under a Commonwealth program, the acronym for which was DIMWITS. I can't remember what it stood for, but having been discharged I now came under the authority of the Repatriation Department.

I studied some Leaving certificate subjects and also commenced a commercial course.

It was a difficult time in many respects. Most of the classes were with young adolescent girls. Sometimes without warning in the quiet classroom, the suction which held my legs on would break with a loud fart-like sound. It was no wonder the girls used to give me a wide berth.

Often, too, climbing the flights of stairs on hot summer days would cause the suction to break, and if I couldn't push my stumps back in, I would have to drag myself on my bum up or down the stairs, then find a private place to put my legs back on. This was done by dropping my pants and putting a sock on my stump and pulling it through a plug in the bucket of the leg. On the odd occasion that some of the young girls saw me doing this, they must have wondered what the hell I was doing.

To make matters worse my English teacher was an anti-war, anti-vet person and we didn't really hit it off.

But I got through and in the New Year presented at the unit that was supposed to oversee my 'rehab', though I had not seen them for the whole year. I was pleasantly surprised when the bloke at the interview said they had kept an eye on me and were pleased with my results. 'Indeed,' he said, 'we have a job for you.' I was elated. We jumped into a car, and he took me to a place not far away. We climbed a set of stairs and entered a workshop. He beamed at me and said, 'Any job here that you want is yours.' I looked around and all I saw were people with intellectual disabilities sitting at benches doing all sorts of menial tasks.

The bastard was offering me a job in a sheltered workshop. I wanted to punch him, but instead left, tears welling as I stumbled back down the stairs. I was devastated, and I swore I would never trust the system again.

But things did change. A friend of my father's was visiting from the eastern states and, unbeknown to me, they went and visited this bloke's mate, who was the officer in charge of the 5th Military District.

A few days later I was invited in for an interview. And a few weeks after that, I had a clerical job working in the army as a civilian. The first pay packet gave me an incredible sense of achievement. It was a small start, but an important one. My wife and I had purchased a modest house with a bit of help from my parents.

We were living in a new suburb in Perth's northern suburbs. I became involved as secretary in the local ratepayers' association and also in my daughter's school P & C (Parents and Citizen's) association. I became heavily involved in the Korea and South East Asia Forces Association of Australia and also with the 'wingies' and 'stumpies' in Perth, better known as the Limbless Soldiers Association. I also joined the local RSL.

I got involved in the local footy and cricket club and, in short, threw myself into life. I was keen to be involved in the community and did not want to be seen to be disabled and useless.

I started to pursue veterans' issues, and in 1975 tried to have the local authority, the City of Stirling, build a memorial to Vietnam veterans. The proposal was vetoed by the mayor at the last minute. The mayor was also a strong member of the RSL and a warden at the state memorial at Kings Park. He argued that individual memorials to individual conflicts would detract from the main state memorial. That response, and a number of other issues, motivated me to run for council. On my first attempt I did not succeed, but on my second attempt I was elected.

The memorial that was rejected in 1975 was eventually built in 1982, and dedicated early in 1983. I left council shortly after, and some years later the mayor who had done so much to stop the memorial was appointed its warden. Life is full of ironies.

I had by now stopped wearing artificial legs. My doctor at Hollywood Hospital, a former gynaecologist, who was in charge of the limb appliance centre, told me I would be forever 'socially incomplete' if I did not wear legs. I had a fair idea by now, however, about what was good for me and what was not.

I used to come home from work with my stumps rubbed raw, bleeding, sore, and uncomfortable. Also because of the height of the amputations, at best my legs would always be cumbersome and severely limiting. I remember one day coming home from work and my wife saying we would need to get someone to clean our gutters of leaves. I took my legs off and dragged a ladder over and climbed the roof and did the job.

Within a few weeks my legs were put down the side of the house and there they stayed. It was the best decision I ever made. I may have been 'socially incomplete' but I was much more mobile, much more comfortable, suffered less from phantom pains, and most importantly for me, was much more independent.

A new job had been advertised which would be a promotion. It was at Hollywood Hospital, and the job description was right up my alley. I applied, did well at the interview, but did not win the job. I was surprised and made a few enquiries. It appeared that the panel was not convinced that I was mobile enough to do the job. My only course of action was to appeal on the grounds of superior efficiency. When I met the panel, however, I spent the whole time convincing them of my mobility and was rewarded with winning the appeal.

Discrimination was alive and well within the public service.

Some time later the Vietnam Veterans' Counselling Service

(VVCS) was opened in Perth, and I was fortunate enough to secure the job as the administration officer. It was an incredible awakening experience for me. Blokes would come into the office and say, 'There's nothing wrong with me, I just want to look around.' But then they would come back again for another look around.

We had two great counsellors at the service, and in time the vets would come in and have an interview. I suddenly recognised in these blokes issues which I had denied in myself: an excessive use of alcohol, feelings of extreme unrest, sleepless nights, depression, anger. Feelings which I had put down to the loss of my legs were being presented on a daily basis by other vets, and I came to recognise in myself what was evident in them: stress disorders. Nowadays these things are better recognised as post-traumatic stress disorder and the VVCS was starting to play an important part in the recognition and treatment of these and other issues being experienced by Vietnam veterans.

I came to appreciate that in many respects I was fortunate. My wounds were plain, evident for all to see. But many blokes who came home from Vietnam carried hidden wounds. Mental health issues not seen were too easily denied by the authorities. Denied and untreated.

I think the Vietnam-era veterans have done more to address these issues than any previous generation of returned soldiers. I shudder when I think of what some of those poor Diggers who came home from the First World War put up with on their return and over the course of their lives.

I had read once where Winston Churchill had written that 'any person who involves him or herself in the community will to some degree or other be drawn toward politics'. And now I found myself so drawn. In 1982 I was approached to stand for the Legislative Council in Western Australia by then Opposition Leader Brian Burke.

I discussed the matter with my wife and within 24 hours decided to have a go. My opponent was a minister in the then government, and no minister in the history of the seat in the Legislative Council had ever been defeated. The swing required was in the double-digit range. So no one was more surprised than I when I won. For me, it was the

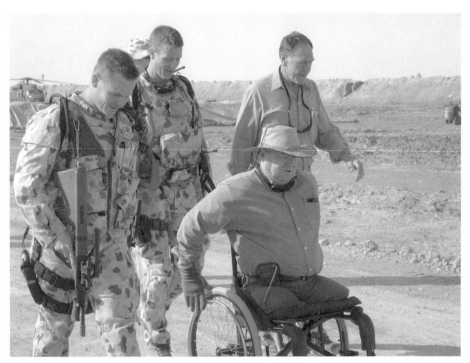

Australian soldiers escort the Honourable Graham Edwards MP to a waiting helicopter at Camp Smitty in Iraq during an inspection tour by Federal parliamentarians, 5 October 2005. Camp Smitty was named in honour of a US Marine who was killed by an improvised explosive device. (AWM P05408.640)

start of an exciting ride. I served for 14 years and had seven years as a minister.

In October 1987, the national Welcome Home Parade for Vietnam veterans was held. After some initial reservations, I decided to attend, and we threw ourselves into a fundraising frenzy in WA to try to get as many vets as possible to Sydney.

It was a wonderful, warm and emotional occasion, and Sydney did Australia and the vets proud. Tears flowed, and years of neglect and ignorance were washed away. Many strong reunions were held by Diggers who had not seen each other for decades. It was an entirely wonderful healing experience. Exactly five years later, in October 1992, came the dedication of the Australian Vietnam Forces National Memorial on ANZAC Parade in Canberra, and this too played an important part in the process of healing and reconciliation for many veterans.

I decided for matters of a personal nature – which I am not sure I still fully understand today – that I wanted to return to Vietnam. In

1970 I had felt convinced I would never want to see the place or the people again.

With a small group of veterans, we went back in 1990 to hold an ANZAC Day service at Long Tan. It was indeed a weird, eerie and confronting experience. When the plane landed, the door opened, and I stared into the eyes of an official in an NVA uniform. I went through something that a psychologist friend of mine later identified as an out-of-body experience. I wondered what the hell I was doing back in the country.

On the afternoon before ANZAC Day, I was asked by then Australian Ambassador to Vietnam, Graham Alliband, to accompany him to a meeting with the local people's committee, who, it appeared, did not want this group of Australians to hold any sort of service at Long Tan.

The meeting was held up a couple of flights of stairs, so I climbed up on my backside and carried my wheelchair with me. Alliband, who was fluent in Vietnamese spoke first; then I said a few words, he interpreted, and the meeting began. It was obviously a hostile meeting. One Vietnamese bloke, in particular, spoke with great passion and emotion and had a lot to say. Alliband and myself were asked to leave, while the meeting continued to deliberate. I was not hopeful that we would have our service.

Waiting outside, I remarked to the Ambassador that the Vietnamese bloke who spoke a lot seemed to be our strongest opponent. Alliband assured me this was not the case. He told me that this bloke, Mr Huy, was a former Viet Cong who had fought against Australians around Nui Dat, and that he wanted us to have the service. He had argued that the committee should let the Australians in, reminding the committee that the Vietnamese would never forget the war, would never forget the loved ones who had lost their lives, and would never forget that it was the Australians who had killed many of them. But, he went on, the war was over, and it was time to look to the future and for the sake of our children and for the Australians' children, we should shake hands and look to becoming friends.

We were permitted to hold our service.

The next day Mr Huy, along with some other former enemy

soldiers, attended the ceremony, and afterwards he invited us to his house for morning tea. I had my old army map with the co-ordinates of my mine incident. He said he knew the area and that he could take me close to the site – but not too close, because there were still active mines in the area.

Huy was indeed a great man, and he became an inspiration to me years later when I decided to run for Federal parliament. I wondered if I would ever have the courage to stand up as he did and argue with his friends and colleagues, advancing a view which he knew to be unpopular and that went against the wishes of his community. I thought he was a man of immense moral courage, and his courage was something I have never forgotten. I met him on subsequent trips to Vietnam, but sadly he has now passed away.

I retired from state parliament in 1996, but following the growth of the 'One Nation' political movement in this country I decided to make a stand and contest a Federal seat. I subsequently won the Liberal-held seat of Cowan in 1998, and entered Federal parliament. I think one of the highlights for me of my time in Canberra was handling the legislation for the Opposition to ban the use of landmines, and I am still the patron for the Australian campaign to ban landmines, though the focus is now on cluster bombs.

The other issue I strongly pursued in Canberra was my passionate interest in veterans' matters. I was always amused – though often angered – in parliament to have successive Ministers for Veterans' Affairs answer questions, or give me a lecture, on how great the system of repatriation is in Australia, and how veterans should appreciate what their government is doing for them. Great patriots these ministers may be, but all they put me in mind of was the bloke who ran the 'rehab' centre in Toorak all those years ago. Australia does have a good system of veterans' affairs, but it is not a great system. A great system would not have let so many veterans fall through the cracks, and it would have done more in previous years to recognise the issue of mental health needs within the veteran community.

I am confident, however, that Defence and Veterans' Affairs are now working collaboratively on issues of mental health – issues denied

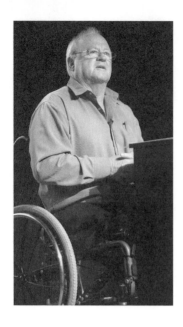

Graham Edwards recounts the moving personal story of his wounding in Vietnam and his experiences of living with his war wounds over the subsequent decades, during the *War Wounds* conference, Australian War Memorial, September 2009. (AWM PAIU2009/141.30)

for so long. But it concerns me that there are still sceptics in authority who fail to believe in issues such as post-traumatic stress disorder. Any soldier who serves in a theatre of war is likely to suffer stress to some degree or other in later years. This can even occur where there is no real danger faced, merely the threat or perception of danger. I know of veterans who served in Vietnam who never went outside the wire and probably faced no real danger. But they faced a threat of danger, and lived their lives with a perception of fear. Because of that experience over a 12-month period, they ran the risk of stress-related mental health issues in later life.

I was recently asked by the Chief of Army to contact a young wounded soldier who had just returned from Afghanistan, where he had lost his legs in an explosion. I decided to go and meet with him. He is a beaut young bloke, keen as mustard to get on with his life. I knew exactly how he felt.

I am very impressed with the manner in which this young soldier is being looked after by the Army. He has been assured that he will be retained in the Army and that he will be given the opportunity to pursue a career and be retrained if necessary. That assurance has given him great confidence. I met with a sergeant from his unit, who has been made his case officer and who also liaises closely with his family.

This young man has been given strong support where years ago that support was non-existent. That sends a clear message to the other Diggers still involved in the war: 'If you are wounded, we will look after you.' I congratulate the Chief of Army for his strong, supportive attitude. It is refreshing and encouraging to know that as the war in Afghanistan continues – and sadly, as the likelihood of further casualties continues – the future security, care and well-being of these young soldiers is paramount in his thoughts. What is also of paramount importance, in the interests of the young men and women who serve in today's ADF, is that the Departments of Defence and Veterans' Affairs (through its Military Rehabilitation and Compensation Commission), work even closer to ensure that no one slips through the cracks. Issues of mental health must be recognised, just as surely as the more visible wounds such as amputation are recognised. These mental health issues must be acknowledged, recognised, and treated.

It is also encouraging and refreshing to know that the treatment many Vietnam veterans received on their homecoming would be unacceptable today. It is true to say that the Vietnam-era veterans leave the veteran community a better place than they found it.

Perhaps I too am a better man for the sum of my experiences. There is, however, not a day that goes by when I don't wish I had legs, and I have to admit that living with war wounds has had its peaks and troughs. My philosophy in life is not whether a glass is half-full or half-empty – rather it is simply if a glass is half-full it is empty. If a life is half-lived, it is wasted. In filling the glass of my life, I know that I have sometimes overfilled it and spilt some. But I also know that I have had a full crack at life and have taken all the opportunities it afforded, opportunities I greatly appreciated made possible by Australians I greatly respected.

I am now over much of the anger that ignited a burning passion within me for so many years. If there is anything I am still seeking today, it is peace of mind and full health. Those qualities I know, however, are as elusive as a politician's promise. I appreciate life and every day lived is a day loved.

I think it is fair to say that I wouldn't be dead for quids.

Notes

Abbreviations used:

AWM	Australian War Memorial (Canberra)
BAB	Bundesarchiv Berlin
IWM	Imperial War Museum (London)
NA	National Archives (Kew, London, formerly PRO)
NAA	National Archives of Australia (Canberra)
NARA	National Archives and Records Administration (US)
NLA	National Library of Australia (Canberra)
PRO	Public Record Office (London, currently NA)
RSL	Returned Services League
USHMM	United States Holocaust Memorial Museum (Washington DC)

Introduction

1 The story of Smith's wounds is recounted in an article by Karen Breslau, 'Healing War's Wounds', in *Newsweek*, 11 September 2006.

2 Kevin Brown, *Fighting Fit: Health, medicine and war in the Twentieth Century*, The History Press, 2008, p. 17.

3 *Ibid.*, p. 37.

4 *Ibid.*, p. 44.

5 *Ibid.*, p. 190.

6 This figure is slightly higher than for Korea because more mortally wounded men were reaching hospital rather than dying on the battlefield.

7 Brown, *Fighting Fit*, pp. 202–3.

8 Many of these injuries stem from the powerful explosives used in the improvised bombs that concuss American troops inside their heavily armoured vehicles. Since 2007, more than 70,000 American service personnel have been diagnosed with brain injuries, ranging from mild to severe. (Source: Associated Press report, 11 November 2009, as reported on http://today.msnbc.msn.com/)

9 Dr Edward V. Craig, 'Wounds of war bring home new ways of healing', 18 March 2008, as reported on http://today.msnbc.msn.com/

10 Anne Underwood, 'War on Wounds', *Newsweek*, 19 May 2008.

11 Simon Gandevia's chapter outlines details of a new award to honour his father's work: the Bryan Gandevia award will be an annual prize to encourage early career historians, particularly those with a demonstrated interest in medical-military history.

Chapter 1

1 In introducing this keynote address to the *War Wounds* conference at the Australian War Memorial in September 2009, Jay Winter opened with the following observation: 'It is right and proper that we speak of a subject of the importance of war wounds here at the Australian War Memorial. This is where serious reflection on the Great War happens. Yours is a unique institution, braiding together the emotive power of a shrine, the representational power of a museum, and the scholarly riches of a great archive. After over 40 years of working in this field, I can say with some confidence that the Australian War Memorial is the premier centre for First World War studies in the world today. It enables scholars and laymen to come together in an act of recognition, the recognition that the Great War shaped the world in which we live.'

2 Anna Akhmatova, 'Why is this century different?', *Selected Poems*, trans. Richard McKane, Bloodaxe Books, 1989, p. 32.

3 On Pat Barker, see Kennedy Fraser, 'Life and letters: "Ghost Writer"', *New Yorker*, 17 March 2009, p. 41.

4 Susan Sontag, 'Looking at war', *New Yorker*, 9 December 2002, pp. 82–98.

5 Paul Weindling, *The Social History of Occupational Health*, Croom Helm, 1985.

6 Jay Winter and Antoine Prost, *René Cassin: Un soldat de la grande guerre*, Fayard, (forthcoming 2010), ch. 2.

7 Paul John Eakin, 'Autobiography, identity, and the fictions of memory', in Daniel L. Schacter and Elaine Scarry (eds), *Memory, Brain, and Belief*, Harvard University Press, 2000, pp. 290–306.

8 Paul F. Lerner, *Hysterical Men: War, psychiatry, and the politics of trauma in Germany, 1890–1930*, Cornell University Press, 1993.

9 Stephen Garton, 'Freud versus the rate: Understanding shell shock in World War I', *Australian Cultural History*, no. 16 (1997–98), pp. 45–59.

10 For instance, see the National Archives, London, PIN 77 files of disabled First World War veterans, a series I established with the help of Professor Bill Nasson of the University of Witwatersrand.

11 On Myers and others, see Ben Shephard, *A War of Nerves: Soldiers and psychiatrists 1914–1994*, Jonathan Cape, 2000, pp. 21ff.

12 Ted Bogacz, 'War neurosis and cultural change in England, 1914–22', *Journal of Contemporary History* (1989), pp. 18–25.

13 On embodied memory, see: A.M. Glenberg, 'What memory is for', *Behavioral and Brain Sciences, XX*, 1 (1997), pp. 1–55; Thomas J. Csordas (ed.), *Embodiment and Experience: The existential ground of culture and self*, Cambridge University Press, 1994; Andrew Strathern, *Body Thoughts*, University of Michigan Press, 1996.

14 See episode 5, 'Mutiny', of the BBC television series I produced in 1996 entitled '1914–18: The Great War and the shaping of the twentieth century'.

15 John Talbott, 'Shell shock and the Second World War', paper presented to 'International conference on the comparative history of shell shock', Historial de la grande guerre, Péronne, Somme, France, July 1998.

16 Martin Eissler, *Freud sur le front des névroses de guerre*, trans. Madeleine Drouin, Presses Universitaires de France, 1992.

17 Lewis R. Yealland, *Hysterical Disorders of Warfare*, Macmillan, 1918; Peter Leese, *Shell Shock: Traumatic neurosis and the British soldiers of the First World War*, Palgrave, 2002; Eric Leed, *No Man's Land: Combat and identity in World War I*, Cambridge University Press, 1979.

18 Samuel Hynes, *The Soldiers' Tale: Bearing witness to modern war*, Allen Lane, 1997.

19 As a start, see: Paul S. Appelbaum, Lisa A. Uyehara, Mark R. Elin (eds), *Trauma and Memory: Clinical and legal controversies*, Oxford University Press, 1997; Cathy Caruth (ed.), *Trauma: Explorations in memory*, Johns Hopkins University Press, 1995.

20 See the special issue of *Journal of Contemporary History*, XXX, 1 (January 2001) on the comparative history of shell shock. See also Mardi J. Horowitz (ed.), *Essential Papers on Post-traumatic Stress Disorder*, New York University Press, 1999; Mardi J. Horowitz, *Stress Response Syndromes: PTSD, grief, and adjustment disorders*, Jason Aronson, 1997; Paul Antze and Michael Lambek (eds), *Tense Past: Cultural essays in trauma and memory*, Routledge, 1996; Yoram Bilu and Eliezer Witztum, 'War-related loss and suffering in Israeli society: An historical perspective', *Israel Studies*, II (1999), pp. 1–31.

Chapter 2

1 The 'rounded' figures quoted are from: John Ellis, *Eye-Deep in Hell: The Western Front 1914-18*, Book Club Associates, 1979, p. 106; A.G. Butler, *Special Problems and Services*, vol. III, *The Australian Army Medical Services in the War of 1914-1918*, 3 vols, Australian War Memorial, 1943, pp. 868, 880; Bill Gammage, *The Broken Years: Australian soldiers in the Great War*, Penguin, 1975, p. 283. As Gammage notes, First World War

statistics are 'notoriously variable'.

2 Peter John Lynch, 'The Exploitation of Courage: Psychiatric Care in the British Army, 1914-1918', Master of Philosophy thesis, University College London, 1977, pp. 110, 114.

3 See: Joanna Bourke, '"Swinging the lead": malingering, Australian soldiers, and the Great War', *Journal of the Australian War Memorial*, no. 26 (April 1995), pp. 10–18; Joanna Bourke, *Dismembering the Male: Men's bodies, Britain and the Great War*, Reaktion Books, 1996, ch. 2; Michael Tyquin, *Madness and the Military: Australia's experience of the Great War*, Australian Military History Publications, 2006, pp. 33–8.

4 For examples, see Richard Holmes, *Tommy: The British Soldier on the Western Front 1914-1918*, Harper Perennial, 2005, pp. 468–71.

5 Dr W. Brown (Wilde Reader in Psychology, University of Oxford; formerly Neurologist, Fourth and Fifth Armies, BEF), evidence in *Report of the War Office Committee of Enquiry into "Shell-Shock"*, His Majesty's Stationery Office (HMSO), 1922, pp. 42–44.

6 Frank Richards (signaller in the Second Royal Welch Fusiliers), *Old Soldiers Never Die*, Anthony Mott Limited, 1983 (first published 1933), pp. 249–50.

7 Keith Simpson, Introduction to Captain J.C. Dunn, *The War the Infantry Knew 1914-1919: A Chronicle of Service in France and Belgium* . . . (published anonymously in 1938), Cardinal, Sphere, 1989, pp. xx, xxv, xxxv; and Appendix by Dunn on the role of the RMO, pp. 585–88.

8 Lord Moran (Sir Charles Wilson, RMO with 1st Battalion Royal Fusiliers), *The Anatomy of Courage*, Sphere Books, 1968, *passim*, especially p. 42.

9 Sergeant R.W. McHenry, 5 Battery, 2 Field Artillery Brigade, AIF, cartoon sketch and caption in rejected contributions for *The Anzac Book*, MSS 1316 box 2; and file 782/64/1,

Australian War Memorial (AWM). For background, see Ashley Ekins, 'A "precious souvenir": The making of *The Anzac Book*', introduction to *The Anzac Book*, Third edition, University of New South Wales Press, 2010, pp. XI–XXXV.

10 Private Cecil Hartt (served with the 18th Battalion AIF on Gallipoli, invalided wounded, AIF HQ London), *Smith's Weekly*, n.d., copy in author's collection.

11 Ashley Ekins, 'Fighting to exhaustion: Morale, discipline and combat effectiveness in the armies of 1918', in Ashley Ekins (ed.), *1918 Year of Victory: The end of the Great War and the shaping of history*, Exisle Publishing, 2010, ch. 7, esp. p. 112.

12 Lieutenant General G.H. Fowke, Adjutant General (AG), GHQ, letter to Judge Advocate General, War Office (WO), London, 12 August 1918, p. 3, WO 32/5484, National Archives, Kew, London.

13 Alistair Thomson, '"Steadfast until death"? C.E.W. Bean and the representation of Australian military manhood', *Australian Historical Studies*, vol. 23, no. 93 (October 1989), pp. 462–78, especially pp. 466–74; Alistair Thomson, *Anzac Memories: Living with the Legend*, Oxford University Press, 1994, pp. 60–72, 145–53; John Barrett, 'No Straw Man: C.E.W. Bean and Some Critics', *Australian Historical Studies*, vol. 23, no. 90, April 1988, pp. 102-14, especially pp. 102–9.

14 C.E.W. Bean, diary, 26 September 1915, pp. 21–34, especially 28–9, 3DRL 606, item 17, AWM 38; extracts quoted in Kevin Fewster (ed.), *Gallipoli Correspondent: The frontline diary of C.E.W. Bean*, George Allen & Unwin, 1983, pp. 156–9.

15 A.G. Butler, *Gallipoli, Palestine and New Guinea*, vol. I, *The Australian Army Medical Services in the War of 1914-1918*, 3 vols, Australian War Memorial, 1938 [first published 1930], *passim*, especially pp. 249–53, 346–50; Butler, *Special Problems and Services, passim*,

especially pp. 75–92, 897, 913, 948.

16 Butler, *Special Problems and Services*, p. 90 n. 53, p. 91.

17 Bean, diary, 14 December 1915, p. 70, 3DRL 606, item 21, AWM 38.

18 Butler, *Special Problems and Services*, pp. 857–63.

19 *Ibid.*, pp. 79–80. Twenty cases of SIW were reported in the single month of October 1915 in the newly arrived AIF 2nd Division, Butler, *Special Problems and Services*, p. 80 n. 37. Butler described the measures taken to control these 'epidemics' and to bring suspected cases to trial. See also Michael B. Tyquin, *Gallipoli: The Medical War: The Australian Army Medical Services in the Dardanelles Campaign of 1915*, New South Wales University Press, 1993, pp. 147–8.

20 Richards, *Old Soldiers Never Die*, p. 50.

21 Dunn, *The War the Infantry Knew 1914-1919*, p. 96.

22 Gammage, *The Broken Years*, pp. 218–19.

23 Ellis, *Eye-Deep in Hell*, p. 112.

24 Gammage, *The Broken Years*, pp. 78–9, 81 n. 99.

25 Major-General Sir Wyndham Childs (Deputy Assistant Adjutant General, GHQ in France, 1914-1916; Deputy Adjutant General, London, 1916-1921), *Episodes and Reflections*, Cassell, 1930, pp. 143–4.

26 Holmes, *Tommy*, p. 61.

27 Niall Ferguson, *The Pity of War*, Allen Lane, Penguin, 1998, p. 367.

28 John Keegan, *The Face of Battle*, Penguin, 1978, p. 275, note.

29 James Brent Wilson, 'Morale and Discipline in the British Expeditionary Force, 1914-1918', unpublished MA thesis, University of New Brunswick, 1978, pp. 59–60, 92–3.

30 Data from *Statistics of the Military Effort of the British Empire During the Great War 1914-1920*, HMSO, March 1922; Bourke, *Dismembering the Male*, pp. 85–6.

31 The data record a total of 126 cases in 1916; 186 in 1917; and 388 in 1918; and a monthly peak of 96 cases in April 1918. A.G. Butler, *The Western Front*, vol. II, *The Australian Army Medical Services in the War of 1914-1918*, 3 vols, Australian War Memorial, 1940, pp. 864–5, Appendix 1 (iv).

32 Butler stated that no Australian statistics were compiled for self-inflicted wounds, but in fact included this data later in the same volume. Butler, *Special Problems and Services*, pp. 90–1, 897, 913 Table No. 42. Bourke misinterprets the total of 700 'reported' self-inflicted wounds as 700 'convictions' for self-inflicted wounds. Bourke, '"Swinging the lead": malingering, Australian soldiers, and the Great War', *Journal of the Australian War Memorial*, no. 26 (April 1995), p. 12.

33 Of the total of 467 courts martial for SIW, 112 cases (25 per cent) were found Not Guilty or Not Confirmed and the defendant was acquitted; 131 cases resulted in sentences of Field Punishment No. 1 and 92 cases in Field Punishment No. 2. Australian courts martial statistics from author's database compiled in the course of a comprehensive study of the complete series of AIF courts martial proceedings files in CRS A471, National Archives of Australia (NAA), completed under conditions of Special Access under the Australian Archives Act.

34 Butler, *Special Problems and Services*, pp. 79–80; Jeffrey Williams, 'Discipline On Active Service: the 1st Brigade, First AIF, 1914-1919', LittB thesis, ANU, 1982, copy, MSS 891, AWM, pp. 40–1; Tyquin, *Gallipoli: The Medical War*, pp. 147–8.

35 2nd Australian Divisional HQ, Circular Memorandum, 'Cases of Self Injury', 28 November 1915, item 229/2, AWM 25; DAG, GHQ, Memorandum, 1 November 1915, item 421/1, AWM 25.

36 Butler, Part 1, *The Gallipoli Campaign*, p. 352.

37 Dr A.F. Hurst (Physician, Nervous Diseases, Guy's Hospital; former officer in charge, Special Neurological Hospital, Seale Hayne), evidence in

Report of the War Office Committee of Enquiry into "Shell-Shock", HMSO, 1922, p. 25. The term 'neurasthenia' was a common broad diagnosis of the various symptoms of soldiers suffering war-related nervous and mental disorders. Peter Leese, Shell Shock: Traumatic Neurosis and the British Soldiers of the First World War, Palgrave Macmillan, 2002, p. 94.

38 Hurst, evidence in Report of the War Office Committee of Enquiry into "Shell-Shock", p. 25.

39 Butler, Special Problems and Services, p. 80 n. 37. Butler here describes the measures taken to control the SIW 'epidemics' and to bring suspected cases to trial. Given the number of cases reported, surprisingly few men were charged for the offence: there were six courts martial for offences committed in October, nine for November, and two for December 1915. Data from author's comprehensive study of AIF court martial proceedings files in CRS A471, NAA.

40 Tyquin, Gallipoli: The Medical War, pp. 147–8.

41 The following case summaries are extracted from the author's comprehensive study of AIF court martial proceedings files in CRS A471, NAA.

42 Manual of Military Law, War Office, 1914, pp. 721–2. Field Punishment No. 1 was a more prevalent sentence within the AIF than is commonly realised.

43 The 18 charges within the AIF for SIW on Gallipoli constituted 3.7 per cent of the total number of SIW charges; 467 (1.3 per cent) of the total AIF charges were for SIW. SIW total 3904 or 1.1 per cent of the total charges in the British Army, Statistics of the Military Effort, Table (xii.), pp. 669–70.

44 Wilson, Morale and Discipline in the British Expeditionary Force, 1914-1918, pp. 143–5.

45 Jeffrey Greenhut, 'The Imperial Reserve: the Indian Corps on the Western Front, 1914-15', Journal of Imperial and Commonwealth History, XII, 1 (October 1983), pp. 54–73, 57. There are some unexplained discrepancies in the statistics quoted by Greenhut, according to Timothy Bowman, The Irish regiments in the Great War: Discipline and morale, Manchester University Press, 2003, p. 45.

46 Santanu Das, 'India and the First World War', Michael Howard (introd.), A Part of History: Aspects of the British experience of the First World War, Continuum, 2008, pp. 63–73, 68. Indian soldiers were subjected to a brutally harsh disciplinary code which included floggings for military offences. The number of death sentences awarded to Indian soldiers, or executions carried out, remains unknown due to the absence of Indian courts martial registers. Gerard Oram, Worthless men: Race, eugenics and the death penalty in the British Army during the First World War, Francis Boutle Publishers, 1998, pp. 103–6.

47 Greenhut, 'The Imperial Reserve: the Indian Corps on the Western Front, 1914-15, Journal of Imperial and Commonwealth History, XII, 1 (October 1983), pp. 60–70.

48 Dunn, The War the Infantry Knew 1914-1919, pp. 311–14.

49 The numbers of recorded SIW cases in the New Zealand Expeditionary Force nevertheless remained comparatively low throughout the war: there were 54 recorded convictions by courts martial, or 2.52 per cent of the total number of 2145 courts martial. Christopher Pugsley, On the Fringe of Hell: New Zealanders and Military Discipline in the First World War, Hodder & Stoughton, 1991, pp. 73–4, 203–4, 347.

50 Butler, Special Problems and Services, pp. 90–1.

51 The available AIF records show that from a total of 700 cases of SIW on the western front (1916–1918), there were 126 SIW cases in 1916, 103 in the period of the Somme battles (23 cases, Apr-Jun; 55 cases, Jul-Sep; 48 cases,

Oct-Dec). Butler, *Special Problems and Services*, p. 913, Table No. 42.

52 Bean, *The Australian Imperial Force in France 1916*, vol. III, *The Official History of Australia in the War of 1914-1918*, 12 vols, Angus & Robertson, 1929, pp. 940–1; Gammage, *The Broken Years*, pp. 174–9.

53 Bean, *The Australian Imperial Force in France 1916*, p. 598.

54 Moran, *The Anatomy of Courage*, pp. 21, 169–70.

55 Bean, *The Australian Imperial Force in France 1916*, pp. 918–21, 925.

56 *Ibid.*, pp. 897–8; Butler, *The Western Front*, pp. 89–90, 515–16.

57 Gammage, *The Broken Years*, p. 174.

58 *Ibid.*, pp. 178–9, 212.

59 Butler, *Special Problems and Services*, p. 913, Table no. 42.

60 Details from author's study of AIF courts martial proceedings files, CRS A471 and soldier's service record file, NAA.

61 There are inconsistencies in the register of the AIF Detention Barracks at Lewes which records that the man was awarded 181 days' detention and served 80 days in prison; 101 days were remitted when he was discharged on 4 August 1919. Item 231/5, AWM 25.

Chapter 3

1 'The Face of Courage,' *Army: the soldiers' newspaper*, Edition 1182, 7 February 2008, p. 2.

2 Arbuthnot Lane, quoted in Elizabeth Haiken, *Venus Envy: A history of cosmetic surgery*, The Johns Hopkins University Press, 1997, p. 31.

3 Carl Ferdinand von Graef quoted in S.L. Gilman, *Making the Body Beautiful: A cultural history of aesthetic surgery*, Princeton University Press, 1999, p. 162.

4 A.G. Butler, *Special Problems and Services*, vol. III, *The Australian Army Medical Services in the War of 1914–1918*, 3 vols, Australian War Memorial, 1943, p. 292.

5 Joanna Bourke, *Dismembering the Male: Men's bodies, Britain and the Great War*, University of Chicago Press, 1996, p. 33.

6 Jay Winter & Blaine Baggett, *1914–18: the Great War and the shaping of the 20th Century*, BBC Books, 1996, p. 364.

7 Gilman, *Making the Body Beautiful*, p. 37.

8 Percy Clare, Imperial War Museum (IWM) 06/48/1, *A Memoir in Four Volumes: Reminiscences 1916–1918*, vol. III. No pagination, undated.

9 *Ibid*.

10 *Ibid*.

11 Reginald Pound, *Gillies: Surgeon extraordinary*, Michael Joseph, 1964, p. 34; Andrew Bamji, 'Facial Surgery: The patient's experience,' in H. Cecil and P.H. Liddle, *Facing Armageddon: The First World War experienced*, Leo Cooper, 1996, p. 492; John Glubb, *Into Battle: A soldier's diary of the Great War*, Cassell Ltd, 1978, p. 192.

12 Anon., *Diary of a Nursing Sister on the Western Front, 1914–15*, William Blackwood and Sons, 1917, p. 47.

13 Tisdall quoted in Lyn MacDonald, *The Roses of No Man's Land*, Michael Joseph, 1980, p. 165.

14 Gillies quoted in Pound, *Gillies*, p. 33.

15 Clare, IWM 06/48/1, vol. III.

16 *Ibid*.

17 *Ibid*.

18 Gillies quoted in Pound, *Gillies*, p. 41.

19 For more on the career of Gillies, see Pound, *Gillies* and Andrew Bamji, 'Harold Gillies: Surgical pioneer,' *Trauma*, vol. 8, 2006, pp. 143–56.

20 Pound, *Gillies*, p. 41.

21 Bamji, 'Facial Surgery,' p. 495.

22 Gillies quoted in Pound, *Gillies*, p. 34.

23 Glubb, *Into Battle*, pp. 185–6.

24 *Ibid.*, pp. 185–93.

25 Letter to the editor, *Lancet*, August 4, 1917.

26 Pound, *Gillies*, p. 42.

27 T.B. Layton, *Sir William Arbuthnot Lane, Bt. C.B., M.S: An enquiry into the mind and influence of a surgeon*, E. & S. Livingstone Ltd, 1956, p. 111.

28 Harold Gillies & D. Ralph Millard, *The Principles and Art of Plastic Surgery*, vol. 1, Butterworth & Co. (Publishers) Ltd, 1957, pp. 38–9.

29 Pound, *Gillies*, p. 42; Pickerill, *New Zealand Dental Journal*, July 1918, quoted in Harvey Brown, *Pickerill: Pioneer in plastic surgery, dental education and dental research*, Otago University Press, 2007, p. 132. For more on the career of Pickerill, see the above biographical work.

30 Tonks in letter to art critic and friend D.S. MacColl, April 1916, quoted in Pound, *Gillies*, p. 30.

31 Daryl Lindsay, *The Leafy Tree*, F.W. Cheshire, 1965, p. 113.

32 *Ibid.*, p. 114.

33 Gillies quoted in Pound, *Gillies*, p. 45.

34 Eric Winter, Sidcup collection – medical records, 1917–1920, Series 96, P3/1/194, Royal Australasian College of Surgeons (RACS), Melbourne.

35 Winter, Sidcup collection, 96 P3/1/194, RACS.

36 Pound, *Gillies*, pp. 55–6.

37 Gillies & Millard, *The Principles and Art of Plastic Surgery*, vol. 1, p. 27.

38 Pound, *Gillies*, p. 35.

39 'Blackie' (Catherine Black), *King's Nurse – Beggar's Nurse*, Hurst and Blackett, 1939, pp. 88–9.

40 Pound, *Gillies*, p. 34; E.D. Toland, *The Aftermath of Battle*, Macmillan and Co. Limited, 1916, pp. 43–4.

41 Gillies & Millard, *The Principles and Art of Plastic Surgery*, vol. 1, p. 45.

42 *Ibid.*, p. 45.

43 Sewell quoted in Pound, *Gillies*, p. 58.

44 Glubb, *Into Battle*, p. 194.

45 Gillies and Millard, *The Principles and Art of Plastic Surgery*, vol. 1, p. 10.

46 *Ibid.*

Chapter 4

1 See Letter to the Inspector-General of the Insane, 3 October 1927, PROV, VPRS 7527/P0001, Unit 1; NAA, B73/56, Box 17, M56846. I have used pseudonyms, where appropriate, to comply with my conditions of access to closed case files.

2 *Ibid.*

3 A.G. Butler, *Special Problems and Services*, vol. III, *The Australian Army Medical Services in the War of 1914–1918*, 3 vols, Australian War Memorial, 1943, p. 880; Department of Repatriation, *Annual Report*, 1938–39, p. 15.

4 'Bedford Park', *RSA Magazine*, September, 1918, p. 51.

5 Jay Winter, *Sites of Memory, Sites of Mourning: The Great War in European Cultural History*, Cambridge University Press, 1995, p. 45.

6 See Roy Porter and David Wright (eds), *The Confinement of the Insane: International Perspectives, 1800–1965*, Cambridge University Press, 2003; Mark Finnane, 'Asylums, Families and the State', *History Workshop Journal*, no. 20, 1985, pp. 134–48; David Wright, 'Family Strategies and the Institutionalised Confinement of "Idiot" Children in Victorian England', *Journal of Family History*, vol. 23, no. 2, 1998, pp. 190–208; David Wright, *Mental Disability in Victorian England: The Earlswood Asylum, 1947–1901*, Oxford University Press, 2001.

7 Roy Porter, 'The Patient's View: Doing Medical History from Below', *Theory and Society*, no. 14, 175–98, 1985, pp. 193–4. Also see Susan Lanzoni, 'The Asylum in Context', *Journal of the History of Medicine and Allied Sciences*, vol. 60, no. 4, 2005, pp. 499–505, p. 499.

8 This literature is extensive. See: Clem Lloyd and Jacqui Rees, *The Last Shilling: A History of Repatriation in Australia*, Melbourne University Press, 1994; Stephen Garton, *The Cost of War: Australians Return*, Oxford University Press, 1996; Michael Tyquin, *Madness and the Military: Australia's Experience of the Great War*, Australian Military History Publications, 2006; Joy Damousi, 'Returned Limbless Soldiers: Identity Through Loss', in *The Labour of Loss: Mourning, Memory and Wartime Bereavement in Australia*, Cambridge University Press, 1999, pp. 85–102; David Gerber (ed.), *Disabled Veterans in History*, University of Michigan Press, 2000; Deborah Cohen, *The War Come Home: Disabled Veterans in Britain and Germany 1914–1939*,

University of California Press, 2001;
Joanna Bourke, *Dismembering the Male:
Men's Bodies, Britain and the Great War*,
Reaktion Books, 1996; Robert Weldon
Whalen, *Bitter Wounds: German Victims
of the Great War, 1914–1939*, Cornell
University Press, 1984; Jeffrey
Reznick, *Healing the Nation: Soldiers
and the Culture of Caregiving in Britain
During the Great War*, Manchester
University Press, 2004; Jennifer D.
Keene, 'Protest and Disability: A New
Look at African American Soldiers
During the First World War', in
Pierre Purseigle (ed.), *Warfare and
Belligerence: Perspectives in First World
War Studies*, Brill, 2005, pp. 215–41;
Jason Crouthamel, 'War Neurosis
and Savings Psychosis: Working-
Class Politics and Psychological
Trauma in Weimar Germany',
Journal of Contemporary History,
vol. 37, no. 2, 2002, pp. 163–82.

9 Butler, *Special Problems and Services*,
p. 965.

10 Limbless and Maimed Soldiers'
Association, 'Improvements
Desired – Pensions and Housing',
20 August 1920, NLA, RSL
Collection, MS 6609, File 701A.

11 See Emily K. Abel, *Hearts of Wisdom:
American Women Caring for Kin*,
Harvard University Press, 2000.

12 Butler, *Special Problems and Services*,
p. 890; L.L. Robson, 'The Origin
and Character of the First AIF,
1914–18: Some Statistical Evidence',
Historical Studies, vol. 15, no. 61,
October 1973, pp. 737–49, p. 739.

13 'The Other Woman's Problems:
Some Intimate Answers to Personal
Queries' Conducted by 'Domina',
Everylady's Journal, 6 December 1917,
p. 748. On the pressure of women
to marry soldiers, see Nicoletta
Gullace, 'White Feathers and
Wounded Men: Female Patriotism
and the Memory of the Great War',
Journal of British Studies, vol. 36,
April 1997, pp. 178–206, p. 191.

14 On women's role in the home see
Kerreen Reiger, *The Disenchantment
of the Home: Modernising the Australian*

Family 1880–1940, Oxford University
Press, 1980, pp. 38 and 39;
'Mothers, Wives and Sweethearts',
Soldier, 22 April 1924, p. 33.

15 See Letter from 'Bitten' in *Duckboard*,
1 May 1926, p. 26; 'Chillblains',
Tassie Digger, July 1921, p. 13;
Record of evidence, 21 March 1929,
NAA, B73/58, Box 80, M15005.

16 Application for Assistance, Centre
for Soldiers' Wives and Mothers,
Mrs Louisa Hogan, 9 July 1917,
NLA, MS 2864, Box 14, File 3.

17 'Mr. Smith, Carlton', typed statement
most likely authored by a Repatriation
Department representative, 1918,
NAA, A2487, 1922/14074.

18 'When the Shell-Shock Soldier
Comes Home', *RSA Magazine*,
June 1919, pp. 19–21, p. 21.

19 Record of Evidence,
Mrs D. Brown, 12 March 1929,
NAA, B73/32, M12490.

20 *Ibid*.

21 See Papers of Harold Kenworthy,
AWM, PR00120.

22 See NAA, B73/37, Boxes 126 and 127,
M74903.

23 Letter to Department of Repatriation,
December 1926, NAA, B73/37,
Boxes 126 and 127, M74903.

24 Undated newsclipping, NAA,
AWM 164. Charles Eyde Berg
died on 30 May 1936.

25 Attachment to letter from
Blinded Soldiers' Association
to Prime Minister, March 1932,
NAA, A461, 0394/1/1.

26 'A Sad Event', *Rutherglen Sun*, 28 May
1918, p. 3. This episode is discussed
in John McQuilton, *Rural Australia
and the Great War: From Tarrwingee
to Tangambalanga*, Melbourne
University Press, 2001, p. 134.

27 Inspector-General of the Insane to
Mont Park Hospital, 16 September
1930, Public Records Office of
Victoria, VPRS 7471/P0001, Unit 3.

28 Letter to the Inspector-General of
the Insane, 3 October 1927, PROV,
VPRS 7527/P0001, Unit 1.

29 Garton, *The Cost of War*, p. 202.
Also see Richard White, 'War and

Australian Society' in Michael McKernan and Margaret Browne (eds), *Australia: Two Centuries of War and Peace*, Australian War Memorial/Allen and Unwin, 1988, pp. 391–423, p. 409.

30 Douglas McMurtrie, *The Disabled Soldier*, MacMillan, 1919, pp. 100, 101.

31 Arnold Lawson, *War Blindness At St Dunstan's*, Oxford Medical Publications, 1922, p. 131.

Chapter 5

1 Callum MacDonald, *The Killing of SS Obergruppenführer Reinhard Heydrich*, Free Press, 1989. For photographs, see Jarolslav Cvancara, Nekomu Zivot, *Nekomuu Smrt 1939–1941*, Laguna, 2002, pp. 335–9.

2 Bundesarchiv Berlin (hereafter BAB) R 31/368. Dr Walter Dick was the doctor praised for treating Heydrich.

3 Peter Witte *et al.*, *Der Dienstkalender Heinrich Himmlers 1941/42*, Christians, 1999, 27 May – 5 June 1942.

4 Keith Mant, *From Nuremberg to the Old Bailey*, ch. 2: 'War Crimes Investigations' (unpublished autobiography); APD (= Leo Alexander Papers, Durham, North Carolina, USA), Alexander to McHaney, 'The Motives of the Sulphonamide Experiments', 5 March 1942.

5 E. Chain, H.W. Florey, A.D. Gardner, N.G. Heatley, M.A. Jennings, Orr-Ewing, Sanders, 'Penicillin as a Chemotherapeutic Agent', *The Lancet*, 2, 1940, p. 226; E.P. Abraham *et al.*, 'Further Observations on Penicillin', *The Lancet*, 2, 1941, pp. 177–88.

6 University Archive (= UA) München E-II-1413 Akten des akademischen Senats der Univ Munchen, AHUB Personal-Akten des o. Professors Karl Gebhardt Bd 1 Sept 1934-43; Hans Waltrich, *Aufstieg und Niedergang der Heilanstalten Hohenlychen (1902 bis 1945)*, Strelitzia, 2001.

7 Alexander Papers Durham, NC (APD) Alexander to McHaney, 5 March 1947 on the motives of the sulfonamide experiments. NARA M

1019/20 Gebhardt interrogation 17 October 1946, pp. 14–19; Gebhardt interrogation by Alexander, 3 Dec. 1946, pp. 19–23. NMT 2/2461 Karl Brandt testimony on 4 February 1947.

8 Harry Marks, *The Progress of Experiment: Science and therapeutic reform in the United States, 1901–1990*, Cambridge University Press, 1997, pp. 100–5.

9 Witte, *Der Dienstkalender Heinrich Himmlers 1941/42*, 7 March, 1 September, 4 September 1941.

10 Paul Weindling, 'Genetik und Menschenversuche in Deutschland 1940–1960. Hans Nachtsheim, die Kaninchen von Dahlem und die Kinder vom Bullenhuser Damm', Hans-Walter Schmuhl (ed.), *Rassenforschung an Kaiser-Wilhelm-Instituten vor und nach 1933*, Wallstein, 2003, pp. 245–74.

11 Imperial War Museum (IWM) Milch diary 26 May 1947; Gitta Sereny, *Albert Speer: His battle with truth*, Macmillan, 1995, pp. 324–5, 387, 409–19, 424–6; Philippe Aziz, *Doctors of Death. Vol. 1 Karl Brandt: The Third Reich's man in white*, Ferni, 1976, pp. 135–9; NARA RG 238 entry 202 box 1 file 3, Friedrich Koch interrogation, 10 March 1947; NMT 12 March 1947 testimony of Friedrich Koch.

12 NARA M 1019/20 Genzken interrogation 20 September 1946, p. 8. AFPB Alexander, 'Questions to be put to Dr. Fischer on the stand', 8 March 1947; PRO WO 309/ 469, A. Martin and Carmen Mory: Report on Carl Gebhardt, 18 Aug. 1945. = NMT 8/ 337; Peter Padfield, *Himmler: Reichs-Führer-SS*, Cassell, 2001, pp. 514, 539, 576.

13 NARA 1019/17 Fischer interrogation by Alexander, 3 December 1946, p. 12.

14 Bernd Biege, *Helfer unter Hitler. Das Rote Kreuz im Dritten Reich*, Kindler, 2000, pp. 173–6; Ernst Gunther Schenck, *Patient Hitler. Eine medizinische Biographie*, Droste, 1989, pp. 475–6; NARA M 1019/20 Gebhardt interrogation 3 December 1946,

p. 29; Ian Kershaw, *Hitler 1936–1945: Nemesis*, Penguin, 2000, pp. 832–83.

15 Reinhard Strebel, 'Das Männerlager im K.Z. Ravensbrück 1941–1945', *Dachauer Hefte*, vol. 14, 998, pp. 141–74, 161.

16 United States Holocaust Memorial Museum (USHMM) Ferriday Papers, box 2, list 22 May 1961.

17 NMT 1019/17 Fischer interrogation 3 December 1946, p. 6; Fischer and Gebhardt statement, 28 December 1946.

18 Mant, 'From Nuremberg', ch. 2: 'War Crimes Investigations'. USHMM Ferriday Collection; W. Woelk, Karen Bayer, 'Herta Oberheuser', *Nach der Diktatur*, Klartext, 2003, pp. 253–68, 261; Alexander, 'Case History of the Polish Witnesses', 17 December 1946, p. 10.

19 NARA M 1019/14 Dzido interrogation.

20 Stanislaw Sterkowicz, 'Medizinische Experimente im Konzentrationslager Ravensbruck', (= Eksperymenty medycne w obozie koncentrazyjnym Ravensbruck), pp. 22–3; NMT 10th Trial Day. 20 December 1946 2/882-3 (re Oberheuser calling them 'Rabbits').

21 NMT 5/109.

22 Freya Klier, *Die Kaninchen von Ravensbrück. Medizinische Versuche an Frauen in der NS-Zeit*, Knaur, 1994.

23 Sterkowicz, 'Medizinische Experimente', p. 21. Germaine Tillion, *Ravensbrück*, Éditions du Seuil, 1973, p. 109; Dunja Martin, '"Versuchskaninchen" – Opfer medizinischer Experimente', Claus Füllberg-Stolberg, Martina Jung, Renate Roebe, Martina Schreitenberger (eds), *Frauen in Konzentrationslagern Bergen-Belsen, Ravensbrück*, Temmen, 1994, pp. 113–22; Martin, 'Menschenversuche im Krankenrevier des KZ Ravensbrück', pp. 99–112; Freya Klier, *Die Kaninchen von Ravensbrück. Medizinische Versuche an Frauen in der NS-Zeit*, Knaur, 1994, pp. 218–21.

24 PRO WO 235/ 305, f. 50 for the BBC broadcast.

25 Tillion, *Ravensbrück*, p. 26.

26 Sterkowicz, 'Medizinische Experimente', p. 21. Klier, *Kaninchen*, p. 257. The delegate was probably Meyer.

27 Martin, 'Menschenversuche im Krankenrevier des KZ Ravensbrück'; Sterkowicz, 'Medizinische Experimente', p. 22.

28 AdeF BB/35/275 Sulfamides – rapport et études, Keith Mant, 'Experiments in Ravensbruck Concentration Camp carried out under the Direction of Prof. Karl Gebhardt', 17 pp. carbon copy no date; Memorandum To Mr McHaney From Major Mant, 5 December 1946.

29 Author's interview with Charlotte Bloch-Kennedy; Paul Weindling, 'The Fractured Crucible: Images of the scientific survival. The defence of Ludwik Fleck', in Johannes Fehr, Nathalie Jas and Ilana Löwy (eds), *Penser avec Ludwik Fleck - Investigating a life studying life sciences*, Ludwik Fleck Centre, Collegium Helveticum, 2009, pp. 47–62.

Chapter 6

1 A transcript of Dimbleby's dispatch of 17 April 1945 for the BBC can be found in Ben Flanagan and Donald Bloxham, *Remembering Belsen*, Vallentine Mitchell, 2005, pp. xi–xiii; and a recording can be accessed at www.bbc.co.uk/archive/holocaust/. A transcript of Murrow's dispatch of 15 April 1945 for CBS can be found at www.jewishvirtuallibrary.org/jsource/ Holocaust/Murrow.html www.archive. org/; and a recording can be accessed at www.archive.org/details/EdwardR. Murrow-BuchenwaldReport.

2 Ohrdruf had been a labour camp, which at its height contained about 10,000 men. Most had been evacuated in the days before the Americans arrived, but the camp remains significant as the first to be liberated with substantial numbers of survivors and the first to be witnessed by the

senior military command. Details (including statistics) about the liberation of the camps can be found in Jon Bridgman, *The End of the Holocaust: The liberation of the camps*, Areopagitica Press, 1990; and Robert H. Abzug, *Inside the Vicious Heart: Americans and the liberation of Nazi concentration camps*, Oxford University Press, 1985.

3 United States Holocaust Memorial Museum Oral interviews. See, for example, liberator Henry Butensky (RG-50.002*31) and survivor Bella Tovey (RG-5-.04260 28).

4 For statistics and detail of the liberation of Belsen see: Imperial War Museum (IWM), *The Relief of Belsen*, IWM, 1991; Ben Shephard, *After Daybreak: The liberation of Belsen, 1945*, Pimlico, 2005; Suzanne Bardget and David Cesarani (eds), *Belsen 1945: New Historical Perspectives*, Vallentine Mitchell, 2006.

5 Jean-Claude Favez, *The Red Cross and the Holocaust*, Cambridge University Press, 1999, p. 271.

6 Paul Weindling, '"Belsenitis": Liberating Belsen, its hospitals, UNRRA, and selection for re-emigration, 1945–1948', *Science in Context*, 19:3 (2006), p. 406.

7 Shephard, *After Daybreak*, represents the first interpretation, while Weindling, '"Belsenitis"' is the revisionist view.

8 There are several excellent studies of the press and the Holocaust. Amongst the best are Barbie Zelizer, *Remembering to Forget: Holocaust memory through the camera's eye*, University of Chicago Press, 1998; and Deborah E. Lipstadt, *Beyond Belief: The American press and the coming of the Holocaust, 1933–1945*, Free Press, 1993.

9 Soviet forces liberated Majdenek, Belzec, Treblinka and Sobibor in July 1944; Auschwitz in January 1945; and Sachenhausen and Ravensbrück in April 1945. These camps had been dismantled or largely evacuated, leaving only a few thousand of the weakest prisoners. In Auschwitz approximately 6000 people were liberated, the vast majority of whom were Jews: about half of them died shortly afterwards.

10 Weindling, '"Belsenitis"', p. 33.

11 Captain R. Barer, Letter dated 2 May, IWM, 93/11/1.

12 See Ben Shephard, 'The Medical Relief Effort at Belsen', in Bardget and Cesarani (eds), *Belsen 1945*, p. 36 and Brigadier H.L. Glyn-Hughes' account of the relief of Belsen to the Royal Society of Medicine, 4 June 1945: British National Archives: WO 222/201.

13 Lieutenant Colonel M.W. Gonin quoted in IWM, *The Relief of Belsen*, p. 22.

14 Papers of Lieutenant Colonel M.W. Gonin, IWM 85/38/1.

15 Papers of Dr A. MacAuslan, IWM 95/2/1.

16 Papers of Dr P.J. Horsey, IWM, Con Shelf.

17 Papers of Dr A. MacAuslan, IWM 95/2/1.

18 Papers of Miss M.E. Allan, IWM 95/8/1.

19 E. Trepman, 'Rescue of the Remnants: The British emergency medical relief operation in Belsen Camp 1945', *Journal of the Royal Army Medical Corps*, vol. 147 (2001), p. 282.

20 Weindling, '"Belsenitis"', p. 403, and Shephard, *After Daybreak*, p. 202.

21 Lieutenant Colonel F.S. Fiddes, Commander No. 10 Casualty Clearing Station, RAMC, Report written August 1945 in the papers of Professor H.C. McLaren, IWM, P435.

22 Major James A. Reed Jr, Investigating Officer, Army Surgeon's Office, 7th US Army, 'Report on the Liberation of Dachau Concentration Camp, 1945', IWM, Misc 154, Item 2384.

23 Papers of Professor H.C. McLaren, then a major serving in No. 10 Casualty Clearing Station, IWM, P435.

Chapter 7

1 I am grateful to Brenda Heagney for comments and corrections on a draft of this chapter.

2 *Australian*, 25 June 1990, p. 9.

3 An Australian War Memorial media release in September 2009 provided details: 'The Australian War Memorial is proud to announce the Bryan Gandevia Award to promote and develop research into Australian military history. A generous bequest by the family and friends of the late Professor Bryan Gandevia has established an annual prize to be awarded to an outstanding postgraduate history thesis in the fields of military or military-medical history. Intended to assist scholars in the early stages of their research career, the prize may also assist with publication of their work. The prize commemorates Professor Gandevia's contribution to the development of Australian military and medical history and to the Australian War Memorial.' (Extract)

4 *Australian*, 25 June 1990, p. 9. Further details of this aspect of the campaign are contained in J. Hooker, *Korea: the forgotten war*, Time-Life Books, 1989, pp. 44–6. See also Darryl McIntyre, 'Australian Army Medical Services in Korea', in Robert O'Neill, *Australia in the Korean War 1950-53*, vol. II, *Combat Operations*, Australian War Memorial and the Australian Government Publishing Service, 1985, ch. 24.

5 B. H. Gandevia, 'Medical and Surgical Aspects of the Korean Campaign, September to December, 1950. Part I. Casualties and their evacuation', *Medical Journal of Australia*, 11 August 1951, pp. 191–5.

6 Soldiers' difficulties in looking after their feet are described in detail in Bryan Gandevia's diary entry for 19 November 1950, PR82/125, AWM.

7 Gandevia's diary of Monday 6 November describes how, because of casualties, he was left 'seriously depleted of trained stretcher-bearers being now six under-strength.' PR82/125, AWM.

8 E.S.R. Hughes and R. Webb, 'Medical and Surgical Aspects of the Korean Campaign, September–December, 1950. Part II. The treatment of open wounds of British Commonwealth battle casualties', *Medical Journal of Australia*, 11 August 1951, pp. 196–8.

9 The typescript of the speech used by the person who introduced Bryan Gandevia is appended to his bound copy of the original *Medical Journal of Australia* article, Gandevia papers, PR82/125, AWM.

10 Gandevia papers, PR82/125, AWM.

11 It was a substantial disappointment to him that his wife's ill health and subsequently his own diminished his academic output, particularly on Australian history.

12 Dr McKenzie became my first PhD student, as we were working on joint research projects at Prince Henry Hospital.

13 B. Gandevia, *An Annotated Bibliography of the History of Medicine in Australia*, Australian Medical Publishing Company, 1956.

14 This is taken from the citation drafted by Dr Brian Billington when Gandevia received a medal from the Royal Australasian College of Physicians in 1988. For some additional detail, see B. Heagney, 'Obituary: Bryan Harle Gandevia', *Health and History*, 2006, 8 (2), pp. 186–91.

15 B. Gandevia, A. Holster and S. Simpson, *Annotated Bibliography of the History of Medicine and Health in Australia*, Royal Australasian College of Physicians, 1984.

16 B. Gandevia, J. Donovan, R. Doust, B. Pribac, B. Proud, R. Travers, *et al.*, (eds), *BIBAM – Bicentenary Bibliography of Australian Medicine and Health Services to 1950*, (4 vols), Australian Government Publishing Service, 1988.

17 B. Gandevia, *Tears Often Shed: Child health and welfare in Australia from 1788*, Pergamon Press, 1978. The release of this book coincided with the first birthday of Sydney's new Prince of Wales Children's Hospital.

18 *Ibid*.

19 B. Gandevia, *Life in the First Settlement*

at Sydney Cove, Kangaroo Press, 1985.

20 M. McKernan, *Here is Their Spirit: A History of the Australian War Memorial 1917–1990*, University of Queensland Press, 1991, pp. 242, 293–6, 317–18.

21 *Ibid.*, pp. 272–4.

22 Apart from the donations to the Australian War Memorial, Gandevia donated most of his books on historical, medical and social history to various libraries and individuals. However, many volumes of his collected medical and social ephemera remain uncatalogued. Since his death in 2006, several key items have been deposited in the Mitchell Library, Sydney. This includes filing cabinets of material previously given to the RACP, containing many reprints, correspondence, memoranda, drafts of papers, extracts from rare books and manuscripts, newspaper clippings, journal extracts, parliamentary papers and reports, graphics and photographs. A 2001 report on this material by Monash University archivist Anne Mitchell states: 'There is no particularly internal order within folders which are often in total disarray due either to reluctance to split files to a manageable quantity of paper or to the creator's habit of extracting material for other purposes, and never replacing it in the original sequence'. The report then focused on 'a few individuals and institutions that have been indispensable to the study of the history of medicine in Australia during the past 50 years. BG is one such and arguably the most influential person of all, whether of his or any other generation.'

Chapter 8

1 I acknowledge the debt I owe the Commanding Officer, Lieutenant Colonel Reg Gardner, the other officers and the men of 4th Field Regiment with whom I served in Vietnam in 1967–68, as well as my colleagues in the Royal Australian Army Medical Corps.

2 J.J. Deller, D.E. Smith *et al.*, *VD in*

Medicine, US Army Internal Medicine, vol. 2, US Government Printing Office, Washington, 1982.

3 J. Tolerton, *A Life of Ettie Rout*. Penguin Books, 1992.

4 B. O'Keefe and F.B. Smith, *Medicine at War: medical aspects of Australia's Involvement in Southeast Asian Conflicts 1950–1972*. Allen & Unwin in association with the Australian War Memorial, 1994, p. 12.

5 O'Keefe and Smith, *Medicine at War*, pp. 387–92.

6 *Ibid.*, p. 399.

7 *Ibid.*, pp. 386 and 391.

8 *Ibid.*, p. 387.

9 *Ibid.*, p. 126.

10 G. Hart, 'Social aspects of venereal disease: I. Sociological determinants of VD', *British Journal of Venereal Diseases*, 1973, 49, pp. 542–7; G. Hart, 'Social Aspects of venereal disease: II. Relationship of personality to other determinants of VD', *British Journal of Venereal Diseases*, 1973, 49, pp. 548–52; and G. Hart, 'Factors influencing venereal infection in a war environment', *British Journal of Venereal Diseases*, 1974, 50, pp. 68–72.

11 Hence the title of my memoir, D. Bradford, *Gunners' Doctor: Vietnam letters*, Random House Australia, 2007.

12 O'Keefe and Smith, *Medicine at War*, p. 103.

13 *Ibid.*, pp. 125–6.

14 G. Hart, 'Factors influencing venereal infection in a war environment', *British Journal of Venereal Diseases*, 1974, 50, pp. 68–72.

15 Bradford, *Gunners' Doctor*, pp. 3, 90.

Chapter 9

1 Source material for this chapter came from papers collected for the publication by Gary McKay and Elizabeth Stewart, *With Healing Hands: the untold story of the Australian civilian surgical teams in Vietnam*, Allen and Unwin, 2009.

2 Letters of Dorothy Angell, private collection.

3 Letter, Dorothy Angell to her family, 15 January 1967, private collection.

4 Dorothy Angell, 'Breaking the Silence: the experience of the civilian nurses in Vietnam', PhD thesis, School of History/Women's Studies, La Trobe University, November 2001.

5 Alister Brass, *Bleeding Earth: A doctor looks at Vietnam*, Heinemann, 1968, p. 21.

6 Interview with Jenny Hunter, S03985, AWM.

7 Interview with Peter Last, S03997, AWM.

8 Interview with Dorothy Angell, F08155, AWM.

9 Interview with Noelle Laidlaw, 25 May 2006, Melbourne.

10 Interview with Von Clinch, S03990, AWM.

11 Interview with Doug Tracy, S03995, AWM.

12 Cablegram, R.L. Harry to DEA, 12 March 1969, file 2481/5/44, A1838, NAA.

13 Interview with Robyn Anderson, S03989, AWM.

14 Interview with Jill Storch, S03980, AWM.

15 The Gold Card enables the holder to access, within Australia, the full range of repatriation healthcare benefits, including choice of doctor, optical and dental care, chiropractic services and pharmaceuticals at the concessional rate.

16 *Commonwealth Parliamentary Debates*, Senate Hansard, 10 November 2000, p. 19727.

Chapter 10

1 Mr Justice Phillip Evatt, *Royal Commission on the Use and Effects of Chemical Agents on Australian Personnel in Vietnam, Final Report*, Australian Government Publishing Service, 1985, vol. 1, ch. IV, p. 21.

2 Repatriation Act 1920 (Amendment Bill 1977).

3 *Commonwealth Parliamentary Debates*, 18 November 1917, Senate, p. 195.

4 Report of the Resolutions, Proceedings and Debates of the Premiers' Conference held at Melbourne, December 1916, in *Commonwealth Parliamentary Papers, Reports of Proceedings of Premiers' Conference, 1916–17*, p. 13.

5 Report of the Resolutions, Proceedings and Debates of the Premiers' Conference (with Ministers of Lands), held at Melbourne, January 1917, (adjourned from December 1916), in *Commonwealth Parliamentary Papers, Reports of Proceedings of Premiers' Conference 1916–17*, p. 9.

6 Minister for Repatriation, Mr Francis, Minister's second reading speech, *Parliamentary Debates*, Australian Soldiers' Repatriation Bill 1943.

7 Clem Lloyd and Jacqui Rees, *The Last Shilling*, Melbourne University Press, 1994 p. 266.

8 Parliamentary debates, Senate and House of Representatives, Commonwealth of Australia, 18 March 1943, pp. 2009-10. Emphasis added.

9 See, for instance, Mr Marwick's exchange with the Attorney-General in Parliamentary debates, Senate and House of Representatives, Commonwealth of Australia, 18 March 1943, p. 1016.

10 The Repatriation Bill 1920 (Amendment Bill 1977) said of the standard of proof: '(2) The Commission, Board, Appeal Tribunal or Assessment Appeal Tribunal shall grant a claim or application or allow the appeal, as the case may be, unless it is satisfied, beyond reasonable doubt, that there are insufficient grounds for granting the claim or application or allowing the appeal.' This is generally referred to as 'reverse onus of proof beyond reasonable doubt'.

11 *Hansard*, Senate, 16 December 1992, p. 5243.

12 Report of the Resolutions, Proceedings and Debates of the Premiers' Conference (with Ministers of Lands), held at Melbourne, January 1917, (adjourned from December 1916), in *Commonwealth Parliamentary*

Papers, Reports of Proceedings of Premiers' Conference, 1916–17, p. 9.

13 The Annual Report of the Veterans Review Tribunal for the year 1983–84 stated that its 'set aside' rate was 13.5% in 1979–80; 34.4% in 1980–81; 66.6% in 1981–82; 87% in 1982–83; and 84.8% in 1983–84. Bruce Topperwien, 'Relaxed Evidentiary Rules in Veterans' Legislation: An empirical analysis', a paper presented at Veterans' Law Conference, Banora Point NSW, 16–17 July 2004 (sponsored by the Veterans Review Board), p. 11.

14 Evatt, *Royal Commission on the Use and Effects of Chemical Agents on Australian Personnel in Vietnam, Final Report*.

15 *Debrief*, Journal of the Vietnam Veterans Association of Australia, vol. 3, no. 19, April 1983, p. 17.

16 Evatt, *Royal Commission*, vol. 7, ch. XIV, Benefits and Treatment, p. 359. See also Topperwien 'Relaxed Evidentiary Rules in Veterans' Legislation: An empirical analysis', p. 11

17 Evatt, *Royal Commission*, vol. 7, ch. XIV, Benefits and Treatment, pp. 364–5.

18 *Ibid.*, p. 366.

19 *Ibid.*, p. 360.

20 *Ibid.*, p. 364.

21 This was the Repatriation Act 1920 (Amendment Bill 1985).

22 'Within a year the amended legislation had led to a rejection of 55 per cent of claims and to a fall in the number of claims lodged or pursued.' Brendan G. O'Keefe and F.B. Smith, *Medicine at War: Medical aspects of Australia's Involvement in Southeast Asian Conflicts 1950–1972*, vol. 3: *The Official History of Australia's Involvement in Southeast Asian Conflicts 1948–75*, Allen and Unwin, 1994, p. 353.

23 Evatt, *Royal Commission*, vol. 4, ch. VIII, Cancer, p. 399.

24 *Ibid.*, vol. 8, ch. XV, Conclusions, Recommendations, p. 22.

25 *Ibid.*, pp. viii, 1.

26 The Royal Commission report identifies two separate standards of proof it is tasked to consider. Of the first it says, 'The Commission adopted the normal civil onus of proof…'. Of the second it says, 'It kept in mind those sections of the Repatriation Act dealing with the standard … of proof required in determinations'. *Ibid.*, vol. 8, ch. XV, Conclusions and Recommendations, p. 10.

27 Administrative Appeals Tribunal, Reasons for Decision: Repatriation Commission v Maree Smith (4/5/1990).

28 Administrative Appeals Tribunal, Reasons for Decision: Humffray v Repatriation Commission (1991).

29 Administrative Appeals Tribunal, Reasons for Decision: Repatriation Commission v Schar (1991).

30 Administrative Appeals Tribunal, Reasons for Decision: Edwards v Repatriation Commission (December 1992); Kain v Repatriation Commission (December 1992).

31 Interviews with Tim McCombe, during March 2009 at the Granville, Sydney, headquarters of the Vietnam Veterans' Federation of Australia. McCombe was the veterans' advocate at many of the Veterans Review Board cases. He also sponsored many of the Administrative Appeals Tribunal cases on behalf of the campaigning veterans.

32 O'Keefe and Smith, *Medicine at War*.

33 Administrative Appeals Tribunal, Reasons for Decision: Repatriation Commission v Maree Smith (4/5/1990); Humffray v Repatriation Commission (1991); Repatriation Commission v Schar (1991); Edwards v Repatriation Commission (December 1992); Kain v Repatriation Commission (December 1992). There were a number of cases which the Repatriation Commission conceded before hearing. There were at least ten such decisions made at the Veterans Review Board in this period.

34 O'Keefe and Smith, *Medicine at War*, pp. 334–5.

35 *Ibid.*, p. 362.

36 *Ibid.*, p. 293.

37 *Ibid.*, p. 362.

38 *Veterans and Agent Orange:* Committee to Review the Health Effects in Vietnam Veterans of Exposure to Herbicides, Division of Health Promotion and Disease Prevention, Institute of Medicine, National Academy of Sciences, National Academy Press, 1993 (prepublication copy).

39 'The committee was . . . conservative in its evaluation of evidence.' Robert MacLennan and Peter Smith, *Veterans and Agent Orange: Health effects of herbicides used in Vietnam*, Department of Veterans' Affairs, September 1994, p. 3.

40 Evatt, *Royal Commission*, vol. 8, ch. XV, Conclusions, Recommendations, p. 22.

41 Robin Hill, 'Old Wounds Re-opened', *Bulletin*, March 15, 1994, p. 41. In the article it is also reported that 'Edwards [the official historian] says he is happy with Smith's contribution'.

42 MacLennan and Smith, *Veterans and Agent Orange*. Professor MacLennan was from the Epidemiology Unit, Queensland Institute of Medical Research. Professor Smith was from the Department of Haematology–Oncology, Royal Children's Hospital, Parkville, Victoria.

43 'At least as likely as not' is equivalent to the Australian civil court standard of 'balance of probabilities'.

44 Evatt, *Royal Commission*, vol. 8, ch. XV, Conclusions and Recommendations, p. 19.

45 *Veterans and Agent Orange: Update 1996*, Committee to Review the Health Effects in Vietnam Veterans of Exposure to Herbicides, Division of Health Promotion and Disease Prevention, Institute of Medicine, National Academy of Sciences, National Academies Press, 1996, ch. 9, p. 17.

46 104th US Congress, 2nd Session, US House of Representatives, Report 104-812. President Clinton, *Announcement by President Clinton, Topic: Agent Orange*, also present: Vice President Al Gore, Admiral Elmo Zumwalt Jr and Secretary of Veterans Affairs, Jesse Brown, Washington DC, Tuesday, 28 March 1996. It became Public Law 104-204 on 26 September 1996.

47 *Veterans and Agent Orange: Update 2008*, Committee to Review the Health Effects in Vietnam Veterans of Exposure to Herbicides (Seventh Biennial Update), Division of Health Promotion and Disease Prevention, Institute of Medicine, US Academy of Science, National Academies Press, 2008, Summary, p. 10.

48 Australian Veterans Health Studies, *Pilot Studies Report*, (4 vols.), Australian Government Printing Service, 1983.

49 O'Keefe and Smith, *Medicine at War*, p. 317.

50 *Morbidity of Vietnam Veterans: A study of the health of Australia's Vietnam veteran community*, vol. 3, Validation Study, Commonwealth Department of Veterans Affairs, November 1999.

51 O'Keefe and Smith, *Medicine at War*, p. 361.

52 Report of the Resolutions, Proceedings and Debates of the Premiers' Conference Held at Melbourne, December 1916, in *Commonwealth Parliamentary Papers, Reports of Proceedings of Premiers' Conference, 1916–17*, p. 13.

Chapter 11

1 I am grateful for information and assistance provided by Hudson Birden (Southern Cross University/University of Sydney), Ashley Ekins (Australian War Memorial) and officials of the Department of Veterans' Affairs. I alone am responsible for the interpretations presented in this chapter, which is an amended and updated version of '"[A] Tangle of Decency and Folly, Courage and Chicanery, but Above All, Waste": The Case of Agent Orange and Australia's Vietnam Veterans', in Graeme Davison, Pat Jalland and Wilfrid Prest (eds), *Body and Mind: Historical essays in honour of F.B. Smith*, Melbourne University Press, 2009, pp. 216–31.

2 Brendan G. O'Keefe and F.B. Smith,

Medicine at War: Medical aspects of Australia's involvement in Southeast Asian Conflicts 1950–1972, Allen & Unwin in association with the Australian War Memorial, 1994. Smith's essay, 'Agent Orange', is on pp. 281–363.

3 A recent example is Graham Walker, 'The Agent Orange story is not over', *Wartime*, 47 (2009), pp. 42–4.

4 Peter Walsh, *Confessions of a Failed Finance Minister*, Random House Australia, 1995, especially p. 28.

5 Smith, 'Agent Orange', p. 361.

6 *Ibid.*, p. 363.

7 Robin Hill, 'Old Wounds Re-opened', *The Bulletin*, 15 March 1994, pp. 40–1.

8 *Ibid.*, p. 41.

9 Committee to Review the Effects in Vietnam Veterans of Exposure to Herbicides, Institute of Medicine, *Veterans and Agent Orange: Health effects of herbicides used in Vietnam*, National Academies Press, 1994. The report is available online at http://books.nap.edu/catalog.php?record_id=2141.

10 Robert MacLennan and Peter Smith, *Veterans and Agent Orange: Health effects of herbicides used in Vietnam*, Department of Veterans' Affairs, September 1994.

11 Minister for Veterans' Affairs, 'Compensation Claims from Vietnam Veterans to be Fast-tracked', media release 118/94, 13 October 1994.

12 'Cassandra' (Peter Walsh), 'Politics and Agent Orange', *Australian Financial Review*, 22 November 1994.

13 E.J. Wilson, K.W. Horsley, R. van der Hoek, *Cancer Incidence in Australian Vietnam Veterans Study*, Department of Veterans' Affairs, 2005.

14 Information from the Commonwealth of Australia Department of Veterans' Affairs.

15 Brian O'Toole, Stanley V. Catts, Sue Outram, Katherine R. Pierse, Jill Cockburn, 'The Physical and Mental Health of Australian Vietnam Veterans Three Decades After the War and its Relation to Military Service, Combat, and Post-Traumatic Stress Disorder', *American Journal of Epidemiology*, vol. 170, no. 3, August 2009.

Chapter 12

1 For a detailed account of this incident, the context of Operation Renmark and the construction of the Viet Cong improvised mine, see Ian McNeill and Ashley Ekins, *On the Offensive: The Australian Army in the Vietnam War 1967-1968*, Allen & Unwin in association with the Australian War Memorial, 2003, ch. 4, especially pp. 115–23.

Chapter 13

1 In the introduction to her presentation at the *War Wounds* conference at the Australian War Memorial in September 2009, Squadron Leader Sharon Cooper delivered the following acknowledgement: 'It is appropriate on an occasion such as this that I give special acknowledgement to the many thousands of personnel who have served Australia and the families who supported them: in particular, those who have paid the ultimate sacrifice in the service of their country and whose names line the walls of the Australian War Memorial. The sacrifice of these brave men and women has guaranteed me the freedom to stand here today and speak of the wounds of war. I share with them all an immense sense of pride and privilege in wearing the uniform of the Australian Defence Force. Lest we forget.'

Index

Page numbers in **bold** refer to illustrations.